The Ministry of Health

Sir Arthur Newsholme

I0894636

Routledge
Taylor & Francis Group

First published in 1925
by G. P. Putnams Sons LTD

This edition first published in 2015 by Routledge
2 Park Square, Milton Park, Abingdon, Oxon, OX14 4RN
and by Routledge
711 Third Avenue, New York, NY 10017

Routledge is an imprint of the Taylor & Francis Group, an informa business

Publisher's Note
The publisher has gone to great lengths to ensure the quality of this reprint but points out that some imperfections in the original copies may be apparent.

Disclaimer
The publisher has made every effort to trace copyright holders and welcomes correspondence from those they have been unable to contact.

A Library of Congress record exists under LC control number: 26000020

ISBN 13: 978-1-138-90518-4 (hbk)
ISBN 13: 978-1-315-69595-2 (ebk)
ISBN 13: 978-1-138-90527-6 (pbk)

Routledge Revivals

The Ministry of Health

First published in 1925, this book explores public health and its administration. It looks at both local and central health administration and surveys the various departments including The Board of Education and The Home Office. The book discusses motives, principles, and results of reform in the sector and gives a history of public health services. Other chapters include those on public health as a career, poor law and public health administration, and health insurance.

THE MINISTRY OF HEALTH

By

SIR ARTHUR NEWSHOLME, K.C.B., M.D., F.R.C.P.

Principal Medical Officer Local Government Board, England and Wales 1908–1919, merged in the Ministry of Health

First Published May 1925

Printed in Great Britain by
THE BOTOLPH PRINTING WORKS
GATE STREET, KINGSWAY, W.C.2

PREFACE

The table of contents which follows this preface shows the general scope of the present volume; but although it has been my privilege to engage in public health work for some forty years, the task of conveying to the socially-minded person a bird's-eye-view of this work has presented serious difficulties.

In such a survey local as well as central administration must necessarily be brought into the picture; and an outline is required of the history of each branch of public health administration, the best guide for the present and the future consisting in a knowledge of the motives and principles of reform, and of the stages by which the present position has been attained.

Fuller knowledge of current health administration is best obtained by taking part in it; and it is in doing this or in steady support of the work of other administrators that the citizen can fulfil his social responsibility.

Some departments of public health administration have been selected for more detailed description. It has been impossible in the available space to detail the important international relationships of hygiene, or to describe in full our national system of vital statistics, which has been an essential factor in promoting sanitary work. The various methods of public education, for the same reason, are left to be inferred from a study of the problems discussed in each chapter. In passing, it may be stated that the most fruitful education is that which can be given to members of parliament and of local governing bodies, to members of the medical profession, and to the many doctors, sanitary inspectors, midwives, health visitors and nurses actually engaged in public health work or in curative medicine. It is through them that a higher standard of hygiene is becoming effective. A properly directed school curriculum can give important help in the same direction.

No attempt has been made, beyond a short statement on the work of voluntary hospitals, to describe the important hygienic work of many voluntary societies, often working through paid agents, in all parts of the country.

Much of our social improvement has had voluntary beginnings, the State lagging behind until the work promised success or its success was demonstrated. To make these experiments and to provide such demonstrations is the chief rôle of voluntary organisations; and the highest good of a voluntary worker is to have his work embodied in an official organisation. This immolation of voluntary work is never complete, for two reasons: first, the official organisation is controlled by elected or co-opted unpaid workers; and second, the transfer leaves the voluntary organisation free to start further social experimentation for the promotion of the communal welfare.

It is too seldom remembered that in this country the vast majority of the total unpaid voluntary workers in Public Health are engaged in official administration, most of them as members of Sanitary Authorities, County Councils, Boards of Guardians, Education Committees and Insurance Committees, many also as Members of Parliament. The last-named are concerned in the ministration of health, by promoting legislation for improved local administration and by critically examining—so far as their limited opportunities and knowledge permit—the administration of the central ministries of health.

Were every Member of Parliament expected to serve a preliminary apprenticeship as a member of one of the local governing bodies of the country, his efficiency in the service of the State would be increased manifold. It is lack of knowledge of local administration in its various branches on the part of our legislators which is largely responsible for the present confusion in local health administration. Again and again, when additional functions were required, and notably in the organisation of National Insurance against sickness, *ad hoc* bodies have been constituted without due consideration of the relation of the new work to that of existing local or central authorities.

It need scarcely be added that for this expression of opinion and for any others in the present volume I am solely responsible. All such opinions are based on long experience of local health administration, followed by eleven years of experience as Principal Medical Officer of the Local Government Board, which then became merged in the Ministry of Health (see pages 25, 96, 103 and 114).

ARTHUR NEWSHOLME.

January 1925.

CONTENTS

CONTENTS

CONTENTS

CONTENTS

THE MINISTRY OF HEALTH

Chapter I

THE HISTORY OF PUBLIC HEALTH SERVICES

I ASSUME for present purposes that the object of public health administration is to conserve and to promote the health of the community by forwarding measures calculated to enhance the general standard of health and by the removal of controllable influences provocative of disease. This being so, it will be appreciated that public health organisation would come somewhat late in the evolution of settled communities. A greater degree of freedom from interruptions by disease became urgent as men aggregated in densely populated towns; but prior to realisation of this urgency, and before means of prevention had been ascertained, two communal provisions were forced on the attention of King and Parliament.

First, there was required protection against marauders, whether inhabitants of the same or of other countries; and so armed forces for offence and defence were an early feature of the life of clan and country; and our police and judiciary system grew up alongside of these armed forces, rendering it possible to discover crime against persons or property and to secure its punishment by a recognised authority. It is a significant fact, however, that a paid police force dates only from the year 1829; and that before that year men subscribed to voluntary societies which made a speciality of tracing and bringing criminals to justice.

Without communal provision for defence against invasion and against criminals, trade and industry could not succeed; and it is at this stage we first meet the problem of compulsion as related to individual liberty, which has important relation to successful public health ministration. Such compulsion can only be successful permanently when it has behind it the continuous will of the majority of the people.

Second, even when a fair measure of freedom from external or intestinal warfare and disorder had been secured, the prosperity of England varied, like that of other countries, with the amount of destitution, whether due to failure of crops or to other causes. Hence arose, more or less cyclically, complex problems of migration, of vagrancy, and of mendicancy, and of more static poverty; and even now with variations of trade and cycles of prosperity and adversity, or on a more limited scale when local or family adversities arise, we see sporadic, or epidemic, or even pandemic poverty, as for instance after the Great War of 1914-18.

It is not surprising, therefore, that from Queen Elizabeth's time onwards special provision has been made for the support of the impoverished at the expense of the rest of the community.

Third, even in mediæval times the nuisances of town life necessitated some elementary sanitary enactments to combat them. The movements of impoverished vagrants and the crowding together of persons who remain fixed to their hovels, especially when associated with malnutrition and with specific poisoning of food and water, have meant, and to a less extent still mean, dangers greater than those of destitution by itself. Disease at intervals became rampant and spread like wildfire, and densely crowded towns—nearly all towns until recently were of this type—were rightly regarded as "graves of mankind"; and in fact their populations were maintained only by rural immigration.

From the preceding sketch it will be evident that the three primary functions of Government are:—

(1) The preservation of law and order, giving safety to life and property.

(2) Protection of the impoverished against the effects of destitution. (The prevention of destitution is a more recent conception.)

(3) Protection against the dirt and filth of human aggregation, which threaten the health of every man, woman and child.

Logically, these three cannot be separated, and in practice they all bear their part in public health administration. The relief of destitution and of its results and its causes, and still more the prevention of destitution form a fundamental public health problem; and running through the whole range of poor law and of public health administration legal enactments to secure compliance with the necessary limitations of individual freedom of action are called for and are enacted. As these enactments are made by the representatives of the people in Parliament and on Sanitary Authorities, their reasonableness is fairly well assured; and the scope and limitations of compulsion in public health work are defined by this condition.

The Evolution of Public Health out of Poor Law Organisation.—Without detailing earlier and more primitive public health regulations and control, which were purely local in their methods of enforcement, it may be said that the earliest public health reforms arose out of Poor Law reforms and are largely associated with the forceful personality of Edwin Chadwick, who was born in 1800. From 1601 the Poor Law had been on a parochial basis; it was hopelessly out of date and full of abuses, when a Royal Commission was appointed with Chadwick as an assistant Commissioner. His indefatigable work in obtaining accurate and first-hand information of the existent evils led to his appointment as a full Commissioner, and the first report of the Commission, dated 1834, introduced Jeremy Bentham's principle of strong centralised control, with a view to securing a uniform degree of efficiency of poor law work. This report also first laid down the principle, regarded as almost inspired wisdom, that the first and most essential condition of relief was that the situation of relieved persons should not become

> "really or apparently so eligible as the situation of the independent labourers of the lowest class."

The motives leading to inquiry into the Poor Laws were not purely economic—alarm at the magnitude of the burden of relief; for almost contemporaneously there was born a sense of communal responsibility for injustice and oppression, and a Factory Commission was appointed in 1833 to consider the shocking condition of children employed in the cotton trade. Among those whose names stand out in humanitarian agitation may be mentioned Richard Oastler, Michael Sadler, and Lord Ashley (Earl of Shaftesbury). The Factory Commission consisted of Mr. Tooke, Dr. Southwood Smith and Mr. Chadwick as Secretary; and without going into detail it is important to note—as bearing on future public health work—that their most important recommendation was in favour of *the appointment of professional paid inspectors*, whose duty it would be to ensure the enforcement of the statutorily limited hours of work of children, their non-exclusion from the benefits of education, and to prevent the public being subjected "to the charges, inconveniences and evils of an ignorant class." This recognition of the need for independent and impartial inspection by officials, representing neither employer nor employed, meant the beginning of a new era in the control of controllable evils, whether of industry, of poverty, or of insanitation; and the intention to secure the schooling of the young workers is no less significant. It was the beginning of the end of the *laissez faire* policy, which, although admirable when first applied to the beneficent release of industry from obstruction to interchange or to freedom of transport, in time became in Chadwick's words a serious evil, for

"as now applied, with the result of letting mischief work, and evils go on which do not affect themselves it is, I consider, a doctrine of revolutionary tendency." *

Inspired, doubtless, from the same source, the Poor Law Commission recommended the appointment of *paid relieving officers* as permanent officials, to undertake the giving of relief on a uniform scale; and Chadwick would have gone further and had complete central governmental control of these officers; but the centralising change was too drastic to be passed, in view of the existence of parochial authorities in each parish.

Probably owing to the non-existence of any local authority to supervise factory control, factory inspectors became, and have remained, officers controlled directly from London.

Some of Chadwick's proposals as to the more systematic classification and segregation of paupers in workhouses have not yet been fully realised; and it is only in recent years that it began to be realised practically that for the old, the sick and for children the principle of deterrence is objectionable.

Under the Poor Law Act of 1834 a Poor Law Board of three Commissioners was appointed, with Chadwick as secretary. Its regulations for controlling local administration were drastic, and much friction arose. Disraeli described Chadwick as a "monster in human shape," and *The Times* regarded the new poor law as "worse than Egyptian bondage." The Board for Englishmen had the fatal defect that it was not directly responsible to an elected body; and in 1847 the Commission was dissolved

* See "The Public Health Agitation, 1833–48." By B. L. Hutchins.

by Parliament, and a Poor Law Board took its place, which was directly responsible to Parliament. Thus it was laid down that responsibility to an elected body is essential for bureaucracy centrally, just as it is to an elected local authority locally. Such limitation by popular control may, and often does, mean interrupted or diminished progress, but the progress made is by consent and is effective, and not subject to the revocals which are liable to affect pure bureaucracy.

But before their disappearance the Poor Law Commissioners had instituted investigations which led directly to the emergence of Public Health organisation. The first visitation of cholera to this country in 1831, which swept off many thousand persons, and the institution of the General Register Office, hastened this. The recording of deaths and their local incidence soon led to the detection of some of the chief centres of excessive mortality. Panic then and subsequently became the parent of sanitation. Although it will be impracticable in these pages to say much more as to our national statistics of mortality—and later of sickness—it is necessary to bear in mind that their publication since 1834 has been a chief driving power of Public Health progress.

In 1834 the Poor Law Commissioners wrote a remarkable letter to the then Home Secretary, Lord John Russell, in which it was stated that

> "The most prominent and pressing of the first class of charges for which some provision appears to be required are for the means of averting the charges upon the poor rates which

are caused by nuisances by which contagion is generated and persons are reduced to destitution. . . . Labourers are suddenly thrown by infectious disease into a state of destitution for which immediate relief must be given. In the case of death the widow and children are thrown as paupers on the parish. The amount of burthens thus produced is frequently so great as to render it good economy on the part of the administrators of the Poor Laws to incur the charges for preventing the evils where they are ascribable to physical causes, which there are no other means of removing. . . .

"We submit to your Lordship the urgent necessity of applying to the Legislature for immediate measures for the removal of these constantly-acting causes of destitution and death. . . . The Board of Guardians have now the services of an efficient body of officers, including experienced medical officers, to guide them in the application of sanitary measures more efficiently than was practicable by the overseers of single parishes under the old system."

It was beginning to be realised that much pauperism in the last resort was due to the wretched housing and sanitation of the poor, and the realisation of this fact led to important reforms which had even deeper influence on the welfare of the people than Poor Law reform or the beginnings of factory reform.

Up to this point we have seen emerge two important reforms:—

(1) The institution of centralised control over

the conditions of work in certain factories, and central supervision with a large measure of control over the work of Poor Law guardians.

(2) The appointment of permanent officials, inspectors and relieving officers, to carry out the newly organised administrative factory and reformed poor law control.

Surveys as Means of Investigation.—Local investigations made on behalf of the Poor Law Board showed the prevalence of "fever" (probably both typhus and enteric fever) and its association with gross insanitation. In one year, of the total recipients of relief in London, one-fifth were the victims of attacks of fever. There followed further surveys, the results of which were embodied in the great "Report on the Sanitary Condition of the Labouring Classes," which showed that

> "such is the absence of civic economy in some of our towns that their condition in respect of cleanliness is almost as bad as that of an encamped horde or an undisciplined soldiery."

These surveys were made by Drs. Arnott, Southwood Smith, and J. P. Kay, and this early appointment of three members of the medical profession to report on the sanitary and social conditions under which the metropolitan poor lived was the first step in the modern utilisation of medicine by the State,* which has now become universal in every district throughout the country, and has been a chief means by which accurate and increasing knowledge has rendered possible the great triumphs of preventive medicine already achieved.

* Simon's "English Sanitary Institutions," p. 185.

Thus in addition to (1) a large measure of centralised control of local work; and (2) the appointment of a paid staff for permanent work, we see the third of the great initial advances towards a Public Health Ministry in the fullest sense of the words, viz. :—

(3) The appointment of medical inspectors for public health inquiries.

With this eventually important development of workers and work, the further general result was established that *an investigation of causes had been contemplated in substitution for alleviation of results ;* and this is the characteristic distinction, up to the present time, between poor law and public health administration.

In one public health matter the medical profession had already been utilised. This arose out of the passing of the Vaccination Act in 1840, which provided that in every parish vaccination at the public cost should be obtainable through the Boards of Guardians. In 1841 it was further enacted that this gratuitous vaccination should not be deemed a disqualifying parochial relief for any public purpose.

A new Royal Commission on the Health of Towns and Populous Places was appointed in 1843 and reported in 1844 and 1845. The evidence had now become too strong for Parliament to ignore. Two temporary Acts, the Nuisance Removal Act and the Disease Prevention Act, were passed, and in 1848 the first Public Health Act was passed, but its operation was limited in the first instance to five years. This Act created a General Board of Health of three members, irresponsible to Parliament, like the Poor Law Board of 1834. Power was given to create Local Boards of Health, and this power was wisely made adoptive, as there was much popular indignation both anent the proposed creations and as to central control. Much ink was spilt in attempts to prove that sanitary regulations were contrary to the rights of the people, while the central control was opposed as unconstitutional, no distinction being drawn between centralisation which decreases local inertia and secures at least a minimum of sanitation, and central meddlesomeness with work adequately in hand.

On the other hand, propaganda then, as now, advocated the new work, the Health of Towns Association, for instance, publishing a weekly sheet of facts and figures.

The General Board of Health survived until 1858; but its independence of Parliament as well as the inevitable unpopularity of its work prepared the way for its destruction; and although its continuance was proposed under a Parliamentary minister, this was rejected, and its work was only allowed to proceed by annual votes from year to year until 1858, when it was dissolved, thus securing a triumph for obstructionists and for those objecting to governmental control of local affairs.

Chadwick himself had resigned from official life in 1855. Simon, while admitting that Chadwick's central control had not always been judicious, bears eloquent testimony to his enlightening work and to his success in first bringing "Health under the Protection of Law."

The more medical functions of the disbanded Board were transferred to the Privy Council by the Public Health Act, 1858, while by the Local Government Act of the same year its other functions were transferred to the Home Secretary.

Much good had been achieved when this unfortunate divorce between expert advice and such attenuated administration as remained took place. Gradually the true relation between filth and disease had become clearer, and there were even glimmerings of the importance of personal as well as environmental hygiene. In 1849 Dr. John Snow pointed the way to specific measures against personal infection by urging—and in 1854 during a later cholera epidemic demonstrating—that cholera is spread by the alvine evacuations of those sick with cholera; and some years later Dr. William Budd established the same point for enteric fever. As years passed the causation of one disease after another was elucidated, and the full importance of avoiding specific contamination of food, milk, and water became realised.

In intensifying the public realisation of the relation between filth and disease and in pressing forward measures for the better organisation of the medical profession and for public health advance, the name of John Simon is pre-eminent. Born in 1816, in 1848 he was appointed the first medical officer of health of the City of London. He at once showed his appreciation of the importance of weekly sickness returns in supplementation of the mortality records of the City, by obtaining information weekly from the poor law medical officers of the City. In the year 1854 the remarkable series of reports made by him to the City Corporation were reprinted in a volume from which the following extracts illustrate the position then occupied by sanitation. Thus in the preface to these reports he states :—

> "The fact is that except against wilful violence life is practically very little cared for by the law. . . . The national prevalence of sanitary neglect is a very grievous fact."

And in these, as in many later reports, he stressed, as needs still to be stressed, the doctrine of responsibility. Thus :—

> "Let not the inquirer too easily admit what will be urged by less earnest persons as their pretext for inactivity—that such evils are inalienable from poverty."

And his outspoken pronouncements on economics should not escape disinterment. Thus :—

> "All labour below this mark (what will purchase indispensable food and wholesome lodgment) is masked pauperism." . . .
>
> "It is the public that, too late for the man's health or independence, pays the arrears of wage which should have hindered this suffering and sorrow."

Again, alluding to the general concurrence of opinion against "any legislative interference with the price of labour," he enters the caveat that the ignorant poor need to be protected, and that the evils of overcrowding, of insanitation, and of adulteration, and so on

> "are not the more to be tolerated for their rising in unwilling Pauperism rather than in willing Filth."

Early Advocacy of a Ministry of Health.—Simon lamented in the same volume that "so completely is our Government dissevered from Science in general, and most of all, from the science relating to life," that there was no tribunal on health matters, and that there was urgent need for the *enforcement* of existing laws, for securing their *progress*, and for their *harmonisation* where discordant.

Referring to the then approaching reconstitution of the General Board of Health, Simon says that the new department whose Parliamentary President he definitely describes as "a Minister of Health,"

> "at least as regards its constituted head, sitting in Parliament, should be, in the widest sense, to care for the physical necessities of human life."

He goes on to say:—

> "Knowledge, and method, and comprehensiveness are wanted—the precise, definite, categorical impulses of a Parliamentary leader, who can recognise principles and stick to them.
>
> "And for such a minister, what a career! It would be idleness to speak of the blessings he could diffuse, the anguish he could relieve, the gratitude and glory he could earn. A heathen can tell him this.
>
> "*Homines enim ad Deos nullâ re proprius accedunt quam salutem hominibus dando.*"

Pursuing our sketch of the progress towards a Public Health Ministry, it is to be noted that in 1847 Liverpool appointed the first local medical officer of health, and the City of London appointed Simon to a corresponding post in the City in the following year. That wide publicity was given to his reports was in part owing to their relating to London; but readers of the preceding extracts from them will rightly attribute their wide publicity chiefly to their caustic and eloquent statement of truths and to the unanswerable cogency and the felicity with which he drove home these truths. A cholera epidemic in 1853-4 again impressed the Government, and in 1855 and for three years afterwards Simon held the post of Central Medical Officer to the General Board of Health. With the transfer of the duties of the General Board of Health to the Privy Council, he held the same post for thirteen years under that body, and for five years subsequently under the newly formed Local Government Board.

I do not propose to follow these see-saw changes. An account of them can be read in Simon's illuminating pages. It suffices to state that although Simon during all but the last five years of his official career was divorced from a share in most branches of administrative control over disease, medical reports were issued from his Department which had great weight in influencing public opinion in favour of more law against and more administrative control over disease; which secured the adequate medical inspection of vaccination done at the public cost; and which produced most important studies on local excesses of disease and on the causes of these excesses.

In 1866 the evidence as to gross insufficiency of the laws for the protection of the public had become overwhelming, and the Sanitary Act of that year was passed, partly under the beneficent stimulus of a current epidemic of Asiatic cholera.

This Act represented an important advance, now justified by the state of public opinion; and to the three great reforms enumerated on page 10 must now be added that, in Simon's words,

> (4) "The grammar of common legislation acquired the novel virtue of the imperative mood," the Act making it the duty of local authorities *to enforce inspection and sanitation of their districts.*

The year 1871 was characterised by a severe epidemic of smallpox and by a menace of a fifth invasion of cholera; and administratively by the issue of the report of the Royal Sanitary Commission which had been sitting since 1869. It had become urgent, in view of the deficiency and entanglements of legislative enactments affecting public health, and the want of system in the sanitary administration of England, that the law and methods of public health administration should be overhauled, and that existing fragmentary and confused sanitary legislation should be consolidated. The Commission made a vitally important recommendation, not even now fully acted on, viz. that "all powers requisite for the health of towns and country should in every place be possessed by one responsible local authority, kept in action and assisted by a superior authority"; or as further expressed in the Report that

> "there should be one authority for all public health purposes in every place, so that no area should be without such an authority, or have more than one."

In places without special statutory constitution it was recommended that the Board of Guardians of each Union should be the public health authority.

So far as central administration was concerned, the Report recommended that

> "the administration of the laws concerning the public health and the relief of the poor should be presided over by one minister . . . which would probably render necessary the appointment under him of permanent secretaries to represent the respective departments."

The Report further declared against centralised local government: "we would leave *direction* only in the central power"; but advised that certain powers of action in default of the local authorities should be conferred on the Central Authority.

It was proposed that all sanitary powers and duties then exercised by other central departments of government should be transferred to the newly authorised Central Board, and that the appointment of medical officers of health should be made obligatory on all local health authorities. These two conditions, which were adopted by Parliament, make it possible to formulate two additional reforms of prime importance, to be added to the four already enumerated (pages 10 and 16).

(5) *Direction rather than control to be the function of the Central Board.*

(6) *Medical watchers over the public health to be universally established in every local area.*

No. 5 conflicts somewhat with No. 1 (page 10), and the two represent the influence of ebb and flow of public opinion as to the proportion between local and central control. The stage now reached meant, in fact, that local authorities—broadly speaking—could be trusted less riskily than in 1858 with the control of their local sanitation.

The reforms thus instituted omitted metropolitan sanitation, the legislative control of the professions of medicine and pharmacy, the control of lunatic asylums, the sanitary regulation of the chief forms of industrial employment, and some other health matters; and therefore, although the new Parliamentary head would be a " Minister of Local Government, he would not, unless he commanded also the other sorts of central sanitary relation, be, in a satisfactory sense, a Minister of Health."*

* Simon.

Chapter II

AN INCOMPLETE MINISTRY OF HEALTH

In 1871 an Act was passed constituting the Local Government Board; and next year an Act amending the constitution and powers of Local Authorities. In 1875 was passed the great consolidating Public Health Act, which even up to the present time remains the chief charter of public health for sanitary districts outside London, though it urgently needs codification with more recent Acts of Parliament and the introduction of amended and extended clauses more nearly in accord with the present stage of development of public health.

It appears desirable to set out as an appendix to this chapter a list of subjects of the chief sanitary clauses of the Public Health Act, for this Act forms the most important landmark in the history of English Public Health. It is impossible here to give a similar list of more recent sanitary enactments, including the numerous Food and Drugs Acts, the Pollution of Rivers Act, the Factory and Workshops Acts, and many others belonging to recent years.

But a few additional remarks on the constitution of the Local Government Board and on the way in which this Board functioned are needed, if the reader is to understand the necessity for the reform which later culminated in the merging of this Board into the Ministry of Health.

In a subsequent chapter the relation of relief of destitution to public health will be further discussed; here we are concerned with a union under one Minister of two functions of Government, which in the earlier years of public health reform were regarded by many as unnaturally united. In practice the combination of poor law and public health activities, in the circumstances and under the conditions in which it became operative, was detrimental to public health interests; and this arose from the preponderant extent to which poor law administration had already become centralised, the poor law guardians in large measure being merely the local agents of the Central Authority, liable to be vetoed on even minute points of local administration.

Simon devotes many pages (348 onwards) to a further cause of inefficiency, which persists to the present day in its main features. It is notorious that the efficiency of the medical services under the Poor Law varies in different areas even now, from a state of lamentable insufficiency and incompetence to one of high efficiency. In the past inefficiency and inadequacy have been the rule; and one reason for this has been that, although through its able general (non-medical) inspectors the Local Government Board has maintained an iron control over the finance and general administration of Boards of Guardians in matters not requiring special hygienic or medical knowledge, the Board always throughout its existence, in Simon's words, "relied very unduly on the sufficiency of non-medical officers in these relations." This has not hitherto been adequately remedied, nor will it be until the medical duties of Boards of Guardians become an intrinsic part of the public health work of the larger local authorities (county councils and county borough councils).

The doctrine—if it may be so called—behind this failure to use expert assistance in the exercise of the drastic and far-reaching powers of the Local Government Board, in matters essentially affecting the health and welfare of the destitute, has been the unbounded faith in "secretarial common sense" (Simon) which reserved medical advice for special occasions, shelving it like a dictionary or cyclopædia for reference, when desired. This is not to state that medical and nursing and hygienic reforms have not slowly infiltrated both central and local poor law organisation; but to state that the process is still far from complete is a mere platitudinous certitude.

The unbounded confidence in glorified common sense in matters of medical and hygienic concern was not the only factor which for long years made the medical care of the sick poor a by-word, and went far to justify the feeling of repugnance of the aged and of mothers of young children to the receipt of poor law relief. An even more potent factor was the great principle of 1834 which enunciated that the position of those relieved must be less agreeable than that of the lowest members of the class from which they come; though there is reason to think that this doctrine when originally formulated was not intended to apply to the sick or to children.

An early mistake in the organisation of the Local Government Board was the appointment of a single chief Permanent Secretary under the Parliamentary President, to be responsible for both poor law and public health affairs. In the then state of opinion that meant the application of poor law methods of supervision, so far as possible, to the new public health duties. Thus the poor law lay inspectors became general inspectors, although destitute of special hygienic and medical knowledge; and it came about that the officers concerned in sanitary work, and especially the medical staff, were relegated to the work of "special consultation and special local inquiries. . . . Thus in respect of administration, the new Office started virtually as a continuance of the old Poor Law Office. . . . The supremacy which had been reserved for secretaries and assistant secretaries in the new office . . . did not give obvious security for the deeper requirements of sanitary administration . . . and implied . . . a dangerously wide discretion or option as to the cases in which skilled advice should be taken . . . and could hardly fail to establish invidious and unsuitable distinctions between inner and outer circles, respectively secretarial and technical, in the sanitary councils of the Board." * And he further says: "The secretariat had been made administrative in as unconditional a sense as if no technical officers existed, or as if mere clerkship was meant to be the Office's sanitary strength."

As decade followed decade the pressure of public health opinion increased; many local authorities

* Simon, *op. cit.*, p. 356.

became stimulant rather than obstructive, and the position of medical officers of the Board approached somewhat nearer, though it cannot be said to have reached, the ideal set out in the following words by Simon (p. 358) :—

> " Reasonable principles (for the Local Government Board) would have been that, so far as the Office was to transact sanitary business, and to deal with questions of sanitary policy, the Secretaries and the Medical Officer should be regarded as one consultative body advising the Minister ; and that delegated powers of action, whether delegated to the Secretariat or to the Medical Officer, should be exercised in the spirit of a joint trust."

To follow the course of public health administration, which steadily improved notwithstanding inadequate and imperfect central supervision and inspection, the reader must be referred to Simon's volume. Improvement was largely associated with the pursuit of special medical investigations by Greenhow, Ballard, Buchanan, Power, and other inspectors or medical officers of the Privy Council and the Board. Gradually the standard of local public health administration became higher, the impetus in this direction originating in the work of local medical officers of health as well as in that of the central medical department of the Local Government Board.

Simon inveighed against the lack of special technical information on variations of local health and administration, arising from imperfect utilisation of the medical staff of the Board and the inadequate numbers of this staff. He particularly alluded to the lack of information as to "the local rates of progress throughout the country in the removal of known causes of disease," and distinguished acutely between accurate scientific information and formal information collected by untrained persons which is little better than a void. An exception occurred in the cholera surveys of ports and riparian districts, though even in regard to these "towards the close of 1886 the unfinished act of supervision was allowed to come to an end, and the previous system of 'how *not* to do it' was tranquilly resumed."

The importance of "keeping some sort of score" of the vital experience of local areas is re-emphasised in various parts of Simon's writings, and the absence of such information is deplored as one of the chief defects in the early history of the Local Government Board. In the history of the Board, and especially from 1890 onwards, many printed reports giving the results of sanitary and epidemiological investigations by medical inspectors let light into dark places, and formed models for local health officers of methods of investigation. The publication of weekly returns of notifiable diseases (see p. 42) and the issue of reports, the deliberate object of which was to bring into the limelight districts with excessive mortality, did much to favour reform. Reference may be made for instance to Dr. S. W. Wheaton's report on the Incidence of Enteric Fever in the different sanitary districts of the county of Durham; and to three reports on Infant and Child Mortality and a report on Maternal

Mortality in the different sanitary areas of England and Wales which were issued from the Medical Department of the Board and which left backward authorities no excuse for making further default in measures to secure improvement. A further important report on Maternal Mortality has recently been issued from the Ministry of Health.

The influence of the Local Government Board in favouring the appointment of satisfactory medical officers of health and in some other matters is incidentally discussed in later chapters.

Before describing the Ministry of Health into which the Local Government Board was merged it will be necessary to set out fully the duties of local sanitary authorities, in other words, the scope of local health administration, and to devote a chapter to the general scope of public health work. The reader will then be favourably placed for forming a judgment as to the sphere of work of a Ministry of Health and its best relation to other central and local authorities.

APPENDIX.

LIST OF CHIEF CONTENTS OF PUBLIC HEALTH ACT, 1875.

Part I. Definitions, &c.

Part II. Authorities for Execution of Act.

Urban and Rural Sanitary Districts.
Description of these.
Powers and duties of Urban Authorities.
Powers and duties of Rural Authorities.
Vesting of Property in Local Authorities.

Part III. Sanitary Provisions.

Sewerage and Drainage.

Sewers vested in Local Authority.
Power to purchase sewers.
Maintenance and making of sewers.
Powers for making sewers.
Sewage to be purified before being discharged into streams.
Alteration and discontinuance of sewers.
Cleansing sewers.
Map of system of sewerage.
Powers of owners and occupiers to drain into sewers of Local Authority.
Power of Local Authority to enforce drainage of undrained houses.
Power of Local Authority to require houses to be drained into new sewers.
Penalty on building house without drains in urban district.
Powers for disposing of sewage.
Power to deal with land appropriated to sewage purposes.
Powers to commence sewage works without district with consent of Local Government Board.

Closet Accommodation.

Penalty on building houses without privy accommodation.
Power to enforce this provision.
As to earth closets.

Privy accommodation for factories.
Public necessaries.
Drains, privies, etc., to be properly kept.
Examination of drains, premises, etc., on complaint of nuisance.

Scavenging, etc.

Local Authority to provide for cleansing of streets and removal of refuse.
Penalty on neglect of Local Authority to remove refuse, etc.
Powers of Local Authority to make By-laws imposing duty of cleansing, etc., on occupier.
Power to provide receptacles for deposit of rubbish.
Houses to be purified, on certificate of medical officer of health or of two medical practitioners.
Penalty in respect of certain nuisances on premises.
Provisions as to cleansing offensive ditches and collections of matter.
Removal of filth on certificate of inspector of nuisances.
Periodical removal of manure from mews and other premises.

Water Supply.

General powers for supplying district with water.
Restriction on construction of waterworks by Local Authority.
As to supply of water.
Power to charge water rates and rents.
Local Authority may require houses to be supplied with water in certain cases.
Powers of water company for supplying water to Local Authority.
Duty of Urban Authority to provide fire-plugs.
Penalty for causing water to be corrupted by gas washings.
Local Authority may take proceedings to prevent pollution of streams.
Power to close polluted wells.

Housing.

Prohibition of new cellar dwellings.
Conditions for use of existing cellar dwellings.
Conditions of registration of Common Lodging Houses.
By-laws to be made by Local Authority.
Sanitary provisions as to Common Lodging Houses.
By-laws as to Lodging Houses.

Nuisances.

Definition of Nuisances.

Duty of Local Authority to inspect district for detection of nuisances.

Local Authority to serve Notice requiring abatement of Nuisance.

Powers of Court of Summary Jurisdiction in dealing with nuisances.

Prohibition in case of house unfit for human habitation.

Power of entry of Local Authority.

Further powers as to nuisances.

Offensive Trades.

Restriction on establishment of offensive trades in urban district.

By-laws as to offensive trades.

Powers of proceeding against offensive trades.

Unsound Food.

Power of medical officer of health and inspector of nuisances to inspect meat and other foods.

Power of justice to order destruction of unsound meat, etc.

Search warrant may be granted by a justice.

Infectious Diseases.

Duty of Local Authority to cause premises to be cleansed and disinfected.

Destruction of infected bedding, etc.

Provision of means of disinfecting.

Provision of conveyance for infected persons.

Removal of infected persons without proper lodging to hospital by order of justice.

Penalty on exposure of infected persons and things.

Penalty on failing to provide for disinfection of public conveyance.

Penalty on letting houses in which infected persons have been lodging.

Penalty on persons letting houses making false statements as to infectious disease.

Powers of Local Government Board to make epidemic regulations.

Hospitals.

Power of Local Authority to provide hospitals.
Recovery of cost of maintenance of patient in hospital.
Power to provide temporary supply of medicine.
Power of Local Government Board to combine Local Authorities.

Mortuaries.

Power of Local Authority to provide mortuaries.
Power of justice to order removal of dead body to mortuary.

The preceding curtailed list gives only the subject of the particular clauses of the Public Health Act, 1875, which are commonly described as "sanitary." Many other clauses have important bearing on public health and efficient local administration.

The subject of some of these is indicated in the following headings:—

Vesting of streets in Urban Authority.
Power to compel paving, etc., of private streets.
Power to purchase premises for improvement of streets.
Power to regulate line of building.
Power to make by-laws respecting New Buildings.
Powers of Urban Authority for lighting their district.
Urban Authority may provide places of Public Recreation.
Urban Authority may provide markets and slaughter-houses.
Every Urban and Rural Authority is required to appoint fit and proper persons to be medical officer of health, surveyor, and inspector of nuisances.
The medical officer of health must be a legally qualified medical practitioner, and the Local Government Board has control over the conditions of appointment and duties of officers, portion of whose salary is paid out of central funds.
Districts may be united for appointing a medical officer of health by order of the Local Government Board.

Chapter III

HEALTH OFFICERS OF LOCAL AUTHORITIES

It is convenient to interpolate at this point an account, however sketchy, of the paid officers who are entrusted with the local executive work of public health administration, as it is chiefly through them that a Ministration of Public Health becomes effective. They are in fact ministers of health, each in his own area of work.

Testimony has already indirectly been given to the valuable work which successive Principal Medical Officers of the Local Government Board, Simon, Seaton, Buchanan, Thorne, Power, have done; to the scientific medical inspections which they have initiated and organised; and to the steadily increasing extent to which their reports, and those of the medical inspectors of the same Board, have influenced the standard of corresponding reports by local medical officers of health. As the last of the Principal Medical Officers of the Board, I can write with authority on the great public value of the reports prepared by the medical inspectors of the Board up to the year 1919, when the Board was merged into the Ministry of Health.

It is a simple statement of fact to record that, owing to the striking improvement in the personnel of the local public health service, there has been a rapid approximation in standard of work of local and central medical officers; and that although the latter are able to focus recent knowledge more successfully than is possible, in most instances, locally; and although the central officers possess more fully the advantage of a wider and a comparative outlook; the relation between the two, always cordial and continuing so, has changed materially as time has passed. This is particularly so in regard to the investigation of local outbreaks of the more common infectious diseases, for which now the local officers seldom require external help. When, however, outbreaks occur reaching beyond the area of a single local administration, and still more in outbreaks of smallpox and typhus and of rarer diseases, help from central medical officers is always welcomed; and in aiding the standardisation of local health administration and in many other particulars their co-operation is invaluable.

The stages by which health officers have reached their present position must be outlined if a satisfactory outlook on current events is to be obtained.

We have seen how the legislature in 1866 made it obligatory on local authorities to arrange for the sanitary inspection of their districts, and to enforce remedial measures as required. In 1872 the legislature made the appointment of medical officers of health and of inspectors of nuisances likewise obligatory in every district. These enactments rendered further sanitary progress possible. The intention of the legislature was that the officer of health should possess expert knowledge not only of medicine but also of its special application to the prevention of disease; and that in the next place, as Simon put it, he should act as "an impartial Public Accuser and Adviser against whatsoever unwholesome influences in his district may be removable under the sanitary law." Evidently such a position involved high moral as well as exceptional professional qualifications. The duties of the post might easily bring the officer into collision with influential persons in his district, such as property owners, butchers and other shop-keepers, and as these and other financially interested persons were often elected on local bodies, the officer's continuance in his appointment might easily be endangered. Evidently, then, from the very first there was risk of failure of this important work unless the officer had security of tenure of his office during the continuance of efficiency, and unless the remuneration for his work was adequate to obviate the need for supplementing his income by private medical practice. An adequate salary from official work could not be obtained in many districts, in view of their smallness and sparse population; and combinations between various districts only exceptionally succeeded. All the duties of rural sanitary authorities were exercised by Boards of Guardians (page 50), and in these areas it was clearly intended that the poor law (district) medical officers, entrusted with the care of the sick poor, should also act as medical officers of health. There was much to be said for this combination. Thus Chadwick in 1842 wrote:—

"It would scarcely be practicable to ensure as certain and well-directed an examination of the residences of the labouring classes, as I conceive may be ensured from the medical officers of the unions."

Simon,* in his first annual report on the "Sanitary Condition of the City of London" (1849), said:—

"I may remind you that each of these gentlemen (having medical charge of the three city unions) works within a certain small and definite district; that he is, therefore, peculiarly competent to speak on the state of the population in that district, on their habits and necessities, on their customary condition of health, and on their liability to epidemic disease; and that the total staff of these officers, taken collectively, representing the medical practice of the whole city, can supply exactly that kind of detailed and precise information which is most serviceable to your officer of health, in guiding him to those more general and comprehensive conclusions which it is his business to lay before you. . . . I am convinced that the expensive and cumbrous proceeding (of obtaining help in sanitary investigation from without) would have a smaller measure of success than that which I submit to you, and which consists essentially in availing ourselves of the local knowledge and daily observations of a staff of officers, already organised and in active occupation for the very purposes in question."

Similarly, Rumsey† (1856) said:—

"There are much higher functions of a preventive nature than those of a mere 'public

* Simon, "Sanitary Conditions of the City of London," p. 62.
† Rumsey, "Essays in State Medicine."

informer' which the district medical officer ought to perform. He should become the sanitary adviser of the poor in their dwellings. Many removable causes of sickness within their own control would be pointed out during his beneficent visits. The miserable effects of alcoholic stimulation might be impressed on the minds of sufferers from intemperance, at times when no warnings or counsels save those of a *medical* visitor would be listened to.

"The state of the apartments of the poor, their clothing and bedding, the choice and preparation of their food, the physical management of their children, their nursing in sickness, would all come occasionally under his cognisance. . . . If the precise cause of mischief were beyond his means of detection, he would direct the attention of the superior officer of health, or the local administrative body, to the matter."

Poor law medical officers visiting the homes of the very poor, and familiar with their home conditions, became part-time medical officers of health. But the attempt to combine prevention and treatment proved unsuccessful, because the poor law medical officers visited only a small proportion of the dwellings of the poor, because they were not trained in preventive work, and because the good seed of preventive work was choked by the increasing competition of private medical practice.

Furthermore, they, like other medical officers of health also engaging in private medical work, did not as a rule possess adequate knowledge of their special health duties. Numerous instances, however, can be quoted of private practitioners acting as health officers who risked their financial interests in the zealous discharge of their public work, and of others in the same capacity who made valuable contributions to the science of epidemiology.

At first, as might be expected, many petty appointments were made, merely giving formal compliance with the law, and presumably this fact determined the subvention or grant which was decided on in the Parliamentary estimates for 1873-4 towards the payment of the salaries of local sanitary officers.

The subject of "Grants in Aid" will again be mentioned (page 111); but it is noteworthy that the Privy Council had prior to this date given two annual subventions: (1) in aid of national education; (2) gratuities to public vaccinators for efficient vaccination, as determined by inspection from the Medical Department of the Privy Council.

The grant now given by the Local Government Board was intended for the payment of one-half of the cost of those local sanitary appointments deemed satisfactory by the Board. (It did not apply to what became subsequently known as county boroughs.) It is unfortunate that this power of the purse, neither then nor in more recent years, has been used adequately to secure good local appointments. Necessarily at first much latitude was necessary. It was a great advance in public health to have secured that in every sanitary area throughout England and Wales there was a medical practitioner having statutory relations with local and (where the grants were received) with the

Central Government, not for treatment of the sick, as in the case of poor law medical officers, but for the prevention of sickness. As time progressed these local appointments, both of medical officers of health and inspectors of nuisances, later renamed sanitary inspectors, became more satisfactory, and statutory provisions were made to secure this.

By the Local Government Act of 1888 County Councils were empowered to appoint medical officers of health; and in another section of the same Act the obligation of sanitary authorities to appoint such officers was conditioned as follows. After January 1st, 1892, no medical officer of health of any district or combination of districts with a population of 50,000 or more shall be appointed medical officer of health unless not only he is legally qualified to practise medicine, surgery, and midwifery, but also unless he has already been a medical officer of health for three years in a district having a population of 20,000, or unless he is registered in the medical register "as the holder of a diploma in sanitary science, public health, or State medicine under section 21 of the Medical Act, 1886."

The conditions under which such a diploma is now given are briefly as follows:—

(1) The candidate must have been medically qualified for two years before he is admitted to the final examination for a public health diploma. The object of this condition is to secure that the candidate shall seriously intend to take up public health work as a career, and that he has had

experience of medical work in a responsible capacity.

(2) The curriculum for the diploma shall extend over at least twelve calendar months during the above-mentioned two years.

(3) The candidate must during at least five months have obtained practical instruction in bacteriology and parasitology (at least 150 hours), in meteorology and climatology in relation to public health (10 hours), in chemistry and physics in relation to public health (90 hours).

(4) The candidate must during at least 80 hours have received instruction in a recognised institution in the principles of public health and sanitation (30 hours), in epidemiology and vital statistics (20 hours), in sanitary law and administration, including public medical services (20 hours), in sanitary construction and planning (10 hours).

(5) The candidate must during three months have attended for two hours on 30 days the clinical practice and received instruction in the method of administration of a recognised hospital for infectious diseases.

(6) The candidate must during six months, and for not less than three hours on each of sixty working days, have been engaged in acquiring a practical knowledge of the duties, routine and special, of a medical officer of health, including all the special services of public health. This experience must have been acquired with a medical officer of health who devotes his whole time to his official duties, or who is in charge of an area having a population of not less than 50,000.

(7) The candidate must pass a satisfactory examination on the above-mentioned subjects, which is divided into two parts.

The possession of this diploma in the vast majority of districts ensures that medical officers of health will be skilled officers, having had a very special training beyond that implied in ordinary medical skill.

So much for their competence. The conditions of their tenure of office have also been greatly improved. The Sanitary Officers Order of 1910 laid it down as a rule that all medical officers of health and inspectors of nuisances, one-half of whose salary is paid from central funds in accordance with section 24 of the Local Government Act, 1884, shall hold office without limit of time until they die or resign, or are removed from office with the consent of the Local Government Board. Under the Public Health (Officers) Act, 1921, and by a later Order of the Ministry of Health, 1922, this security is further extended. Metropolitan and county medical officers of health have security of tenure of office by separate statutory enactment. In all cases provision is made for determination of office for misconduct, insanity, etc.

Next to security of tenure, an adequate salary and a retiring pension—which is in substance merely deferred payment—form important inducements for competent physicians to devote their life to public health work. No arrangements can be regarded as satisfactory which do not give the medical officer of health a good status among the general practitioners in his district, and which do not avoid the shadow of poverty after his retirement. In recent years steady improvement in these respects has occurred. The Local Government and other Officers Superannuation Act, 1922, renders it possible for local authorities, other than Boards of Guardians, to adopt the scheme for superannuation embodied in the Act. This scheme, when adopted, involves the contribution by officers holding established posts of 5 per cent. of their salaries, the local authority contributing an equal amount, the superannuation thus secured being equal to one-sixtieth for each year of service of the average salary received during the five years immediately preceding the date of retirement. Many local authorities have already adopted this Act, and will thus undoubtedly be aiding the efficiency of their staff, both by securing a better class of recruits and by enabling officers to retire at the age of 65.

The duties of the medical officer of health are complex and necessitate a very varied training. He must have administrative capacity and tact in the management of men and affairs; a full and sympathetic knowledge of social conditions is most helpful; and he must have a logical mind, competent in the sifting of evidence. An adequate knowledge in clinical medicine and special skill in diagnosing doubtful attacks of infectious diseases are essential. As the communal physician, the guardian of health of the public, he must have scientific knowledge of all influences favouring health or undermining it.

The Local Government Board and the Ministry of Health have laid down a list of the chief duties of the medical officer of health, which are as follows, in the words of the official order, or summarised from this :—

(1) He shall inform himself as far as practicable respecting all influences affecting or threatening to affect injuriously the public health within the District.

(2) He shall inquire into and ascertain by such means as are at his disposal the causes, origin, and distribution of diseases within the District, and ascertain to what extent the same have depended on conditions capable of mitigation or removal.

(3) He shall by inspection of the District, both systematically at certain periods, and at intervals, as occasion may require, keep himself informed of the conditions injurious to health existing therein.

(4) He shall advise the Council on matters affecting the health of the District, and give certificates for legal purposes.

(5) On receiving information of the outbreak of any infectious or epidemic disease of a dangerous character within the District, he shall visit without delay the spot where the outbreak has occurred, and inquire into the causes and circumstances of such outbreak, and in case he is not satisfied that all due precautions are being taken, he shall advise the persons competent to act as to the measures which appear to him to be required to prevent the extension of the disease and shall take such measures for the prevention of disease as he is legally authorised to take under any Statute in force in the District or by any Resolution of the Council.

(6) Subject to the instructions of the Council,

he shall direct or superintend the work of the Inspector of Nuisances in the way and to the extent that the Council shall approve, and on receiving information from the Inspector of Nuisances that his intervention is required in consequence of the existence of any nuisance injurious to health, or of any overcrowding in a house, he shall, as early as practicable, take such steps as he is legally authorised to take under any Statute in force in the District, or by any Resolution of the Council, as the circumstances of the case may justify and require.

(7) In any case in which it may appear to him to be necessary or advisable, or in which he shall be so directed by the Council he shall himself inspect and examine any animal, carcase, meat, poultry, game, flesh, fish, fruit, vegetables, corn, bread, flour, or milk, and any other article to which the provisions of the Public Health Acts in this behalf apply, exposed for sale, or deposited for the purpose of sale or of preparation for sale, and intended for the food of man, which is deemed to be diseased, or unsound, or unwholesome, or unfit for the food of man; and if he finds that such animal or article is diseased, or unsound, or unwholesome, or unfit for the food of man, he shall give such directions.

(8, 9 and 10) He shall perform all necessary duties as to by-laws and inquire into offensive processes of trade, and attend at the office of the Council as required.

(11 and 12) He shall report his proceedings to the Council and the measures which may require to be adopted for the improvement or protection of the public health in the District; also as to the

sickness and mortality within the District. He shall also keep records.

(13) He shall send to the Ministry of Health a weekly return of the cases of infectious disease notified to him during the preceding week.

(14) He shall make an annual report on the sanitary circumstances, the sanitary administration, and the vital statistics of the District.

(15) He shall report forthwith to the Ministry of Health any case of Plague, Cholera, or Smallpox or of any serious outbreak of epidemic disease in the District which may be notified to him, or which may otherwise come to his knowledge.

The duties of the Sanitary Inspector are set out in the same Order. He acts, subject to the instruction of the Council, under the general supervision of the medical officer of health, and his duties are closely related to those of that officer. He must furnish annually to the medical officer of health a tabular statement showing—

(*a*) The number and nature of inspections made by him during the year.

(*b*) The number of notices served during the year, distinguishing statutory from informal notices.

(*c*) The result of the service of such notices.

The medical officer of health is the administrative head of the local public health department; and is administratively related to all the special officers in this department. He has intimate links also with other officers concerned in public health matters who may not be technically within his department.

With the *Public Analyst* of Foods and Drugs

occasional consultations are necessary, in order that the character and variety of samples for analysis may be decided, and in order that the sanitary inspector charged with this work may have competent guidance. Similar remarks apply to the *laboratory pathologist*, concerned in examining suspected material from cases of tuberculosis, venereal disease, typhoid fever, diphtheria, etc. With *medical practitioners* engaged in general practice a cordial relationship is necessary to ensure success in public health work. The following rules have been found useful in practice :—

(1) Encourage consultations about doubtful cases of infectious disease, however irksome this may be.

(2) Avoid differences of opinion in the presence of relatives. Isolation rooms at the Fever Hospital often supply a way out of the difficulty of such cases.

(3) Take every opportunity to explain the fallacies of negative pathological returns, and offer assistance in taking specimens in certain cases.

The medical officer of health may also have important relations with practitioners undertaking part-time work in school clinics or tuberculosis clinics or child welfare centres, or in venereal disease clinics; and while respecting their clinical independence he is responsible for the general system followed in any clinic paid for out of official funds.

The chief officers with whom he may have almost daily consultations are :—

(1) Sanitary inspectors.
(2) Health visitors.
(3) Tuberculosis nurses.
(4) School nurses.

In larger areas his contact will be chiefly with the medical heads of each of these sub-departments, his work consisting chiefly in the general organisation of each special branch of work and in ensuring that there is close co-operation between each of these.

The medical officer of health is responsible also for general oversight over the work of the Fever Hospital, the Smallpox Hospital, the Tuberculosis Dispensary, Sanatorium and Hospital, and any other Hospitals, or Hospital Beds, e.g. for convalescent or crippled children, that may be subsidised by the Council.

The scheme given on page 55 illustrates well the complexity of the duties of a medical officer of health of a large town.

It is evident therefore that the Annual Report of the medical officer of health, which is in substance an annual stocktaking, requires to be a comprehensive document. The following items are required to be included in it either annually or in fuller detail every fifth year. In addition to any other matters upon which he may consider it desirable to report, his Annual Report shall contain the information indicated in the following paragraphs; together with such further information as the Ministry of Health may from time to time require:—

(*a*) An account of any influences threatening the health of the District, the prevalence of infectious or epidemic diseases therein, and the measures taken for their prevention.

(*b*) An account of all general and special inquiries made during the year.

(*c*) An account of the work performed by the Inspector of Nuisances during the year, including the statement supplied in pursuance of Article XX (16) of this Order.

(*d*) A statement as to the conditions affecting the wholesomeness of the milk produced or sold in the District.

(*e*) A statement as to the conditions affecting the wholesomeness of foods for human consumption, other than milk, produced or sold in the District.

(*f*) A statement as to the sufficiency and quality of the water supply of the District and of its several parts, and in areas where the supply is from water-works, information as to whether the supply is constant or intermittent.

(*g*) A statement as to the pollution of rivers or streams in the District.

(*h*) A statement as to the character and sufficiency of the arrangements for the drainage, sewerage and sewage disposal in all parts of the District.

(*i*) A statement as to the privy, water-closet, and other closet accommodation in the District, including information as to the approximate number of each type of privy and closet.

(*j*) A statement as to the character and efficiency of the arrangements for the removal of house-refuse, and the cleansing of earth-closets, privies, ashpits, and cesspools in the District.

(*k*) A statement with regard to the housing accommodation of the District as required by Article V of the Housing (Inspection of District) Regulations, 1910, and an account of any other action taken by the Council under the Housing,

Town Planning, etc. Act, 1909, bearing on the public health.

(*l*) A statement as to the vital statistics of the District, including a tabular statement, in such form as the Ministry of Health may from time to time direct, of the sickness and mortality within the District.

(*m*) Where the Medical Officer of Health is appointed by the Council of a County Borough, or by a Council having delegated powers under the Midwives Act, 1902, a statement as to the administration of that Act in the District.

The subjects requiring to be stated in a complete Annual Report will include :—

(*a*) A description of the natural and social conditions of the District, including occupations, conditions as to poverty, hospital and other relief, overcrowding, etc.

(*b*) A statement of the chief sanitary circumstances as to—

(1) Water supply.

(2) Rivers and streams.

(3) Drainage and sewerage.

(4) Closet accommodation.

(5) Scavenging.

(6) Sanitary inspections of District.

(7) Premises controlled by special ordinances, e.g.:

Lodging-houses.
Offensive trades.
Cellar dwellings.
Slaughter-houses.

(8) Schools.
Details of sanitary conditions.
Details of medical inspections.
Details of arrangements for treatment.

(9) Food, including milk.
Details as to avoidance of adulterations and contamination.
Inspection of cows, cowsheds and dairies.

(10) Housing inquiries under the Housing Acts.

(11) Inspection of workshops, shops, etc.

(*c*) Sanitary administration.

(1) Work of staff.
Sanitary inspectors.
Health visitors.
School and tuberculosis nurses.

(2) Details of work under (*a*) and (*b*).

(3) Administration of hospitals.

(4) Administration of special ordinances.

(5) Work in public health laboratories.

(*d*) Prevalence of and control over Acute Infectious Diseases.
Statistical information in tabular form.
Information as to sources and methods of spread.
Methods of control.

(*e*) Prevalence of and control over Tuberculosis.
Statistics of deaths and notifications.
Report of Tuberculosis Officer, including information on Dispensaries, Sanatoria, sanitary visiting, etc.

(*f*) Prevalence of and control over Venereal Diseases.
Report by medical officers of clinics.
Propaganda, etc.

(*g*) Investigation of other diseases.
Special industrial diseases of the district.
Prevalence of Rickets, Pneumonia, Acute Rheumatism, etc.

(*h*) Maternity and Child Welfare.
Statistics of infantile and maternal mortality.
Puerperal sepsis.
Administration of Midwives Act.
Infant and pre-school consultations.
Home visiting.

(*i*) Relation of Official to Voluntary Workers.

(*j*) Vital statistics of the District.

The Annual Report is not merely a stocktaking record intended for the local Council and the Ministry of Health. It should comprise remarks for reading by the public; and as time passes there is happily an increasing public who are keenly interested in a clear summary of existing defects not yet remedied, in a general statement of progress made, and in instruction and advice on current health subjects.

The wise medical officer of health does not report continuing defects as though these constituted a personal grievance; but with courtesy and consideration, always remembering that progress in matters of popular government necessitates the education of a majority to his own way of thinking, and that progress made as the result of this is permanent, even though only partial. From this standpoint it often happens that in administration the best is the greatest enemy of good.

Although the medical officer of health necessarily is the chief officer in the local Public Health Department, this does not detract from the value attaching to the indispensable work of the Sanitary Inspector and the Health Visitor. The work of the last-named is sketched in Chapter XVI. That of the *Sanitary Inspector* calls for some further remarks at this point. His statutory change of title from that of Inspector of Nuisances gives the key to his advancing importance. He, like the medical officer of health, is now less concerned with the *abatement* of nuisances and disease-producing conditions, and more with their *prevention.* He is expected to possess special qualifications and to have had careful training, as evidenced by a special certificate of competency obtained from special examination boards. He is responsible for the extremely important work of inspection of dwellings under the Public Health Acts and the Housing and Town Planning Acts. He has important duties in regard to inspection of foods, and the collection of samples for detection of adulteration. In respect of many of the matters of pure sanitation, indicated on pages 26 to 28, he is the chief officer concerned. He receives and investigates complaints as to nuisances, as to factory smoke, etc., and is responsible for advising as to the removal of nuisances and for giving evidence when notices to abate nuisances have not been complied with.

No history of Public Health would accord with experience which did not give Sanitary Inspectors a high position in the successful battle which has been waged against the various forms of insanitation.

Chapter IV

LOCAL MINISTRATION OF HEALTH

Local administration for purposes of health and for the avoidance of nuisances was at first concerned with the removal of excremental matter, human or animal, from the neighbourhood of houses, and with such patent nuisances as pig-keeping near to human dwellings. Hence in earlier Sanitary Acts, clauses relating to privies, to pig-keeping, to scavenging, and the duties of inspectors of nuisances are prominent; and it must not be supposed that the importance of such matters has diminished.

In the following scheme are shewn the chief Central Authorities concerned in the health of the people, and their relation—if any—to local health authorities. In this chapter the work of Local Education Committees (see p. 132) and of Local Insurance Committees (p. 199) is not considered.

It will be seen that there are 144 larger Public Health Authorities (County Councils 62, and County Borough Councils 82). More or less affiliated to the County Councils and having statutory public health connection with these there are

29 Metropolitan Borough Councils,
253 Municipal Borough Councils,
782 Urban District Councils, and
663 Rural District Councils,

SCHEME OF CHIEF LOCAL AUTHORITIES CONCERNED IN HEALTH IN RELATION TO CENTRAL AUTHORITIES.

I
Ministry of Health.

(a) Public Health Authorities.

Each geographical county comprises an administrative County and (with few exceptions) county boroughs. The Authorities concerned are

- County Councils (62)
  - Metropolitan Borough Councils (29)
  - Municipal Boroughs (253)
  - Urban Districts (782)
  - Rural Districts (663)
- County Borough Councils (82)

(b) Poor Law Authorities.

Poor Law Unions occasionally overlap into two counties. There are 635 Boards of Guardians.

(As a rule these do not coincide with sanitary areas.)

(c) Local Insurance Committees.

62 for county areas and 82 for county borough areas.

II
Board of Education.

(d) Local Education Authorities (Education Committees).

Each geographical county comprises an Administrative County, County Boroughs and smaller Education Authorities as follows.

- County Council Education Areas (62)
- County Borough Education Areas (82)
- Other Boroughs and Urban Districts (173)

III
Home Office.

No special local organisation, but M.O.H. and Sanitary Inspector have certain limited duties as to Factories and Workshops.

Also industrial diseases are notified by local medical practitioners to H.M. Inspector of Factories, Home Office. (As to certifying surgeons see page 120.)

making altogether 1,727 Public Health Authorities, as compared with 317 Education Authorities and 635 Boards of Guardians. In addition there are Parish Councils exercising some minor sanitary functions.

The chief difficulty in efficient sanitary administration is the existence of an excessive number of small sanitary areas.

The following statement from my evidence before the Royal Commission on the Poor Laws (Appendix, Vol. ix) shows the allocation of population in poor law unions and in urban and rural sanitary districts. It may be taken as approximately applying at the present day.

> "Taking the country as a whole, the average population of sanitary areas is not much more than one-third that of unions. This is owing chiefly to the number of very small urban and rural sanitary districts. Of the total 660 rural districts and 1,129 urban districts 8.5 per cent. of the former and 19.9 per cent. of the latter had a population under 3,000, 18.4 per cent. of the former and 39.1 per cent. of the latter had a population under 5,000, 52.4 per cent. of the former and 62.2 per cent. of the latter had a population under 10,000. On the contrary, only 12.7 per cent. of the Poor Law unions had a population under 10,000. These figures need to be partially qualified for the few districts which have combined to secure the services of a medical officer of health who devotes the whole or a large part of his time to the public service. Such combined authorities do not affect materially the

general view that more than half of the sanitary authorities—happily, however, representing a much smaller proportion of the population of the country—consist of units of less than 10,000 population.

"Experience has shown that, as area of administration is sub-divided below certain minimum limits, so local personal interests predominate; and that, in accordance with this, a very large proportion of the smaller sanitary authorities are unworthy of their powers. Local considerations of expense and favouritism, and the insecurity of tenure of office of their sanitary officers, make efficient work an exception. A chief reason why sanitary progress has been impeded, is furnished by the continued existence of these unsatisfactory small sanitary authorities. They do not as a rule obtain skilled advice, nor can they afford to obtain it when uncombined with other districts. Even when such advice is obtained, a small area of administration increases the risk of its neglect.

"In considering, therefore, the work of sanitary authorities under any improved conditions, it is indispensable that the anomalously small authorities must be combined or re-distributed into units of at least the same order of magnitude as that of the large majority of the parochial unions, so that each may have within the reasonable limits of its purse the minimum staff and equipment required for efficiency."

Since the above comments were made combination of areas for the work of the medical officer of health has occurred more frequently; but this does not secure the satisfactory administration which could be obtained by complete fusion of the sanitary authorities concerned. What is required is that the number of sanitary authorities should be reduced to one-third their present number, the smaller number, outside county boroughs, being related to public health administration on a county scale. The following table from a paper written by me in 1909 showed for that date—and some of the anomalies persist—the excessive cost of sanitary supervision in the areas having ridiculously small populations.

The cost of the sanitary services as indicated by the salaries of medical officers of health and of inspectors of nuisances in each of the subjoined groups of districts is stated in the following table in terms of the population served by £1 of salary given under each head:—

In districts having a population.	No. of population served by £1.	
	With Medical Officer of Health.	With Inspector of Nuisances.
Under 2,500	95	58
2,500-5,000	144	110
5,000-10,000	197	97
10,000-15,000	237	127
15,000-20,000	218	150
Over 20,000	197	213
In boroughs	191	184
In county boroughs	446*	?

* Some county boroughs have also assistant medical officers of health.

Evidently the expenditure stated in proportion to population is heaviest in the smallest districts. In such areas, as remarked in my Annual Report to the Local Government Board (1907-8, p. viii)

> "Local self-government is both extravagant and inefficient. There is an unnecessary multiplication of officers, who cannot be paid sufficiently to devote themselves without distraction to the public interests; on the part of the sanitary authorities of paltry districts like these, local and personal considerations too often outbalance the public interests, and the multiplication of small areas is a serious obstacle to an efficient and economical settlement of problems of water supply and sewerage in which neighbouring districts are mutually concerned."

It is scarcely necessary for our purpose to describe in detail the functions of each form of sanitary authority, but the general character of these duties is partially shown in the list of the sanitary clauses of the Public Health Act given on page 25; and a further clue is furnished by the statement in the last chapter as to the duties and annual reports of medical officers of health.

In the following summarised statements the chief items of work of the Public Health Departments of a County Borough Council and of a County Council are enumerated :—

A. A Large County Borough.

Infectious Diseases.—Investigation. Fever Hospital. Disinfection. Cleansing Station. Provision of anti-toxin.

Laboratory Work for infectious diseases, etc.

Maternity and Child Welfare.—Home visiting by Health Visitors. Infant Welfare Centres. Antenatal Clinics. Educational work. Maternity beds. Convalescent Homes. Observation wards for sick children. Clinics for massage and remedial exercises. Day nurseries. Provision of milk and meals. Dental treatment. Investigation of still-births, puerperal fever, ophthalmia neonatorum. Supervision of midwives.

Tuberculosis.—Investigation of notified cases. Home supervision and nursing. Dispensary. Sanatorium. Hospital. Shelters. Case work. Bacteriological work. X-rays. Drugs, foods, and apparatus.

Venereal Diseases.—Clinics. Drugs. Laboratory work. Educational work.

Mental Deficiency.—Statutory and school cases. Occupation centres.

School Medical Service.—Medical inspection in elementary and secondary schools. Clinics for minor ailments (ringworm, eye, throat, ear, dental, massage, remedial exercises, breathing). Following up of defective children. Medical work in special schools for physically and mentally defective children, and in Open Air Schools. Orthopædic schemes. Cleansing. Provision of milk or meals. Examination of teachers, nurses, etc. Investigation of infectious and contagious diseases.

Blind Persons Act.—Ascertainment, care and employment schemes.

General Sanitation.—Investigation of complaints. Nuisances, including smoke. Inspections of premises. Fly prevention. Offensive trades.

Housing.—Inspections on complaint, and house to house. Service of notices. Drain testing. Houses let in lodgings. Common lodging houses. Sanitary surveys.

Food Inspection.—Cowsheds. Dairies. Milk shops. Slaughter-houses. Butchers. Grocers. Greengrocers. Bakehouses. Ice-cream manufacturers. Hotel and restaurant kitchens, etc. Sampling under Food and Drugs Acts. Markets and Street Trades.

Factories, Workshops and Workplaces.—Inspections. Out workers.

Shops Acts.—Inspections.

Other.—Rat extermination. Work under Rag Flock Act and Fertilisers. Cinemas, etc. General administration.

B. A County Council.

Infectious Diseases.—Ascertainment of sufficiency of hospital accommodation for smallpox and other infectious diseases.

Laboratory Work in some areas.

Maternity and Child Work.—Home visiting by health visitors. Infant Welfare Centres. Antenatal clinics. Maternity Beds. Provision of milk and meals. Dental treatment. Investigation of still-births, puerperal fever, ophthalmia neonatorum. Supervision of midwives.

Tuberculosis.—As in A.

Venereal Diseases.—As in A.

Mental Deficiency.—As in A.

School Medical Service.—As in A.

Blind Persons Act.—As in A.

Housing.—General supervision of housing

accommodation in the administrative county, but without any large direct powers.

Food and Drugs Acts.—Sampling, etc. in some areas.

Pollution of Rivers and Streams.—Inspection. Remedial powers.

Water Supplies.—Inspection. Remedial powers.

Other.—Rat extermination. General consultation work. General administration.

The method of working of a Borough Council may be taken as an example of the mixed voluntary and official agents employed. For a borough of say 200,000 persons, the Town Council—the local Parliament for the chief varieties of public health work in the borough—may have about 40 councillors and 15 aldermen, one-third of the former being subject triennially to election by the ratepayers of their respective wards. The Mayor of the town is elected annually. He has no special powers, except as chairman of the Council. The detailed work of the Council is dealt with by various committees each consisting of about 12-15 councillors and aldermen, the mayor being *ex officio* a member of every committee. The chief committees usually are the following:—

General Purposes,
Finance,
Police,
Health (Housing may be dealt with by a separate Committee),
Education,
Roads, Sewers and Constructions,
Maternity and Child Welfare,
Education.

The chief officers of the Corporation (not including commercial undertakings such as the supply of electricity, gas, tramways) are the

Town Clerk,
Medical Officer of Health,
{Surveyor and Engineer,
{Architect,
Accountant,
Chief Constable,
Education Officer,
Waterworks Engineer,

who may be called on by any Committee of the Council for expert advice, and who systematically attend all meetings of the committees most closely related to their special work. It is in these committees that the expert officer and the representatives of the people on the Council exchange views, and proposals are subjected to exhaustive discussion and criticism. The Chairman of the Committee is responsible for putting before the entire Council special proposals of any Committee, the official not being heard as a rule in the public meeting. This arrangement works well. The expert officer has an adequate hearing in committee and by means of formal written reports; and, even when his proposals are "turned down" or accepted in an attenuated form, he has the satisfaction of knowing that progress when made is solid and satisfactory, and not liable to reaction and interruption. In these respects his position compares very favourably with that usually occupied by medical and other technical advisers in various Government Departments.

Local Councils can make by-laws regulating

housing, lodging-houses, offensive trades, slaughter-houses, etc., subject to approval of the draft by-laws by the Ministry of Health, and these by-laws then have the force of law. Apart from these the powers of local government, as a rule, extend only to what is expressly and specifically authorised by Parliament. Their administrative powers are wide, their legislative powers very limited. To meet this restriction large municipalities have frequently applied to and received from Parliament extended powers in particular branches of public health work; and such extensions subsequently are commonly given to other local authorities applying for them. In this way an additional valuable body of sanitary legislation has accumulated, some of which has become incorporated in general law, and some waits to be so incorporated.

Notwithstanding the limitation of local autonomy, associated with the absence of local legislative powers, the work of our municipalities is of even greater importance than that of the legislature: for while the latter may enact suitable laws, it is on the consistent and persistent action of the former that a high standard of sanitary administration depends.

Two obstacles to efficient sanitary administration urgently wait to be remedied.

(1) There is needed a general overhaul of our local sanitary areas and abolition of all the smaller units of administration, these being merged into larger units. The work done in these smaller units is inefficient, both parsimonious and extravagant, besides being liable to the favouritism which in larger units is greatly checked.

(2) The formation of larger units with more comprehensive duties would assist in removing the lack of local patriotism now commonly evidenced by failure of ratepayers to vote at local elections, thus giving corruptly interested persons the opportunity to get elected. Some part of this lack of interest in local government arises from the greater mobility of population associated with the increasing trend towards urban and suburban life. Our large towns are encircled by "dormitory" suburbs and villages, the inhabitants of which seldom interest themselves in local government. This "delocalisation" of a large part of the inhabitants may mean that the control of local affairs falls into the hands of people with axes to grind, unless a band of social workers by persistent vigilance prevent this.

Voluntary social welfare societies foster local patriotism; and in addition local administration is strengthened by the co-option of a certain number of non-elected persons on to the Education Committee and the Maternity and Child Welfare Committee of a local authority, thus enabling the local authority to obtain the help of persons having special knowledge of the work in hand.

In local government as in central government the guiding principle—subject to the exception indicated on page 94 is that there should be one and only one local authority for all purposes in which health is concerned; and for efficiency all the smaller sanitary authorities should be merged into larger authorities.

It may be accepted that an important function of the Ministry of Health in relation to the work of the local authority should be the formulation of *a minimum standard of sanitation*, and there should be only a limited amount of inspection of work done by aid of Government grants, always subject to the ensurement of the attainment of a minimum standard of work in each special branch of work for which grants are given. These special branches of work are considered in chapters xvi–xviii. Meanwhile the following may be regarded tentatively as the main points in ordinary public health work, for which a minimum standard is required.

(1) Adequate sanitary arrangements for every family.

(2) Satisfactory separate water supply for every family.

(3) Accommodation for every family supplying at least one room for every two persons.

(4) Adequate and satisfactory storage of food and of fuel.

(5) Provision for the supply of domestic hot water.

(6) Access to medical treatment and nursing for all below a certain rental.

(7) Adequate hospital provision, general and special.

Special local services are described in subsequent chapters, including the Insurance and Destitution Services, all of these being connected centrally with the Ministry of Health.

At this stage, before considering the functions of the Ministry of Health, prior remarks on the relation between central and local authorities and on the general distribution of governmental functions appear to be needed, if one is to avoid confusion in considering the best methods and machinery of public health administration. And prior even to this some preliminary remarks on the possible scope, and some of the results so far obtained from, public health work are desirable.

Chapter V

THE SCOPE OF PUBLIC HEALTH WORK

In preceding chapters the scope of public health work has already been roughly indicated, as was inevitable, in our sketch of Public Health Advance, including the history of the Local Government Board, and of the rapid evolution of the medical officer of health as a servant of the public health. The sketch in the last chapter of current local public health administration has shed additional light on the present activities of sanitary authorities.

There is needed at this stage, however, a more general view of the still undeveloped and in some respects unexplored possibilities of further improvement which will be rendered possible when an efficient central Ministry of Health has associated with it reformed local health authorities. As a preliminary to this it is desirable to indicate the statistical evidence of improved national health between the formation of the Local Government Board in 1871 and its merging into the Ministry of Health in 1919. For this purpose I give here a summary of remarks which formed part of my Annual Report for 1917-18 as Principal Medical Officer to the Local Government Board.

1871-1919.

There has occurred an immense improvement in

health and duration of life since the Local Government Board was formed in 1871, and the work of local sanitary authorities became more completely organised. This statement is no reason for contentment, but rather an incitement to increased effort towards extensions of public health and medical work and the simplification of administrative machinery needed to this end.

The establishment of the Local Government Board represented a real advance in public health development, by concentrating in one department of the central government the supervision of local government, and especially of such local government as related to the public health and the relief of the poor.

The progress secured may be partially measured in terms of reduction in national mortality; and this reduction is strikingly illustrated in a statement by Simon in his first report as medical officer of the Local Government Board. In this report he stated that the approximately half million deaths a year from all causes then occurring in England and Wales were a third or about 125,000 more numerous than they would be if throughout the country existing knowledge of the chief causes of disease were reasonably applied. In my annual report for 1917-18, I stated that the 514,879 deaths occurring in 1871 would have been reduced by 200,000 had 1871 shared the average national experience of the period 1911-15; and the improvement secured in recent years is further illustrated in the following table:—

England and Wales.

Average Annual Death-rate per 1,000 *living at each age period in* 1911-15

Ages.											
0–	5–	10–	15–	20–	25–	35–	45–	55–	65–	75–	85 & upwards
36.7	3.4	2.1	2.9	3.5	4.5	7.4	13.3	27.0	58.6	131.8	262.9

Percentage reduction of Death-rate when 1911-15 *is compared with* 1871-80.

Ages.											
0–	5–	10–	15–	20–	25–	35–	45–	55–	65–	75–	85 & upwards
42	48	43	46	51	50	42	25	15	10	7	15

It will be seen that up to the age period 45-55 the death-rate has declined from 42 to 51 per cent.; and that even at higher ages there has been a substantial reduction of the death-rate. Stated in terms of life-table experience, there has occurred in the experience of males an increase in the average expectation of life at birth of ten years, and in the experience of females of nearly eleven years, when the experience of 1871-80 is compared with that of 1910-12. Furthermore more than 70 per cent. of this increased duration of life in males has occurred at ages 15-65, the most useful years of life.

Enteric fever furnishes perhaps the most important index of sanitary progress; and the course of events indicates that it may safely be anticipated that in not very remote years this disease will become almost as rare in this country as is typhus fever. Typhus fever has been eradicated by the prompt and general isolation of those suffering from it, by limiting the movements of those incubating the disease, by clearing out rookeries in our cities, and by the greater cleanliness of the population, thus diminishing the scope of action of body-lice by which the disease is spread. With steadily increasing protection of water supplies, adequate supervision and control of milk supplies, the abolition of conservancy methods of excrement disposal, the more complete enforcement of protective measures against the consumption of contaminated shell-fish, and the recognition of "carriers" and the adoption of precautionary measures regarding them, enteric fever is now similarly a rapidly disappearing disease. The progress in the prevention of enteric fever already secured is shown in the following figures :—

England and Wales.

In 1871, with a population of 22⅘ millions, 12,709 deaths from enteric fever occurred.

„ 1881	„	„	26	„	6,688	„	„
„ 1891	„	„	29	„	5,200	„	„
„ 1901	„	„	32⅗	„	5,172	„	„
„ 1911	„	„	36⅕	„	2,430	„	„
„ 1916	„	„	34½	„	1,137	„	„

Since 1911 the cases of enteric fever in the whole country have been tabulated in annual returns prepared in the Medical Department of the Local Government Board. The rapid decline of cases of enteric fever since that date is shown below.

ENGLAND AND WALES.

In 1911 the number of cases of enteric fever notified was ..	13,852
„ 1912 „ „ „ „ ..	8,386
„ 1913 „ „ „ „ ..	8,263
„ 1914 „ „ „ „ ..	8,445
„ 1915 „ „ „ „ ..	6,364
„ 1916 „ „ „ „ ..	5,564
„ 1917 „ „ „ „ ..	4,601

The almost complete disappearance of typhus fever and the gradual vanishing of enteric fever can fairly be regarded as due to public health administration during forty years. The lowered general death-rate is only attributable in part to this cause, but it is certain that general improvement in sanitation in its widest sense has borne an important part in reducing both respiratory and diarrhœal diseases, and in causing the reduced prevalence of tuberculosis. Its influence is also shown in reduced prevalence of many other diseases.

It should be noted that the immense improvement experienced in the prospects of health and life has occurred in face of the adverse influence of increasing urban aggregation, with its devitalising influences and its multiplied opportunities for transmission of catarrhal and other infections. In 1871, 61.8 per cent., and in 1911, 78.1 per cent. of the total population of England and Wales were living in urban districts.

Improved conditions of life have gone far to counterbalance the evils of urban life; and among the influences conducing to this end the work of sanitary authorities and their sanitary officers stands high. A pure water supply, improvements in food supply, more adequate scavenging, drainage and sewerage, the clearing out of courts and alleys, better housing (that housing has greatly improved does not mean that further improvement is not greatly needed), street paving and sanitation have all helped. So likewise have the improvements in industrial hygiene, especially in the prevention of industrial dust and the reduction of hours of labour. These factors have been greatly aided by the steadily improving education of the people, and by the preventive work of police authorities and voluntary agencies, especially in regard to drunkenness and cruelty to children; and it is certain that the improved material comfort of the population with a rising standard of feeding and clothing has played a large part.

Quoting from the exact words of the above-mentioned report, it should be added that

> "The improvement resulting from the above complex social and sanitary causes has had to be paid for; and the rapid growth of local rates and of loans of local authorities is made the subject of occasional lugubrious warnings. In so far as these warnings help to secure provident spending on well-considered schemes of reform they are valuable. Local expenditure has ofttimes been mistakenly incurred. This is a reason for wiser guidance in the future, not for the extravagant parsimony which refuses to spend what is needed to secure the highest obtainable standard of communal health and welfare. On the whole, allowing for extravagances and blunders, the results achieved by local authorities justify

the expenditure incurred, with the warning that combination of smaller authorities is needed to avoid in the future redundant small schemes and liliputian administrative arrangements.

"In the year 1871-2 the total local taxation expenditure in England and Wales was officially given as £31,185,471; in the year 1911-12 the total aggregate expenditure of all local authorities (other than expenditure defrayed out of loans) was given as £134,073,327. In 1871-2 the outstanding loans of all local authorities amounted to £69,461,087, in 1911-12 they were £556,571,139. Of the 134 millions expenditure in 1911-12 roughly 30 millions was for education, 15 millions for highways, bridges, etc.; 12 for poor-law relief, including institutions; 8 for police and justice; 4 for asylums; 2 millions for isolation hospitals; 4¾ millions for electric lighting; and 7¾ millions for gasworks; waterworks nearly 6 millions; sewerage nearly 5 millions; tramways nearly 9 millions, etc. Against many of these items receipts for services rendered need to be balanced.

"More than a quarter of a million fewer persons die annually than would die if the experience of the decennium, 1871-80, continued. This implies an enormous annual saving of sickness and disability, of loss of wages, of the production of dependent widows and orphans, etc. One of the chief causes of poverty is sickness. The greater part of such poverty is outside the scope of the poor-law organisation; but within its range it is known that about 30 per cent. of paupers are sick, and according to the estimate of the Royal Commission on Poor Laws 'at least one-half of the total cost of pauperism is swallowed up in direct dealings with sickness,' to which, of course, must be added the indirect expenditure on those impoverished by the sickness of wage earners or house-wives."

1919-1924.

To complete the preceding review it is desirable briefly to indicate the further improvement in vital statistics since the Great War ended. The figures for the war period 1914-18 are abnormal, and can only be utilised in respect of infant mortality and enteric fever.

In respect of infant mortality the war period 1914-18 was marked by events which influenced child health favourably. A large proportion of the fathers were away from home, but liberal allowances were made to the mothers, and there was a great increase in the activity of maternity and child welfare workers (page 208). Their efforts were doubtless greatly helped by the fact that the war period was one of greatly reduced alcoholic consumption throughout the country.

The general course of events during a series of years is shown below :—

Infant Mortality (under one year) per 1,000 *Births.*

1901–5 ..	138	1916–18 ..	95
1906–10 ..	117	1919–21 ..	84
1911–15 ..	110	1922–23 ..	74

The more recent course of *Typhoid or Enteric Fever* has been as follows :—

In 1918 the number	of cases	of enteric	fever	notified was	..	4,232
„ 1919	„	„	„	„	..	3,308
„ 1920	„	„	„	„	..	2,994
„ 1921	„	„	„	„	..	3,776
„ 1922	„	„	„	„	..	2,365
„ 1923	„	„	„	„	..	3,139

The total standardised death-rate from all causes has steadily improved, except during the influenza pandemic of 1918. In 1913 it was 13.5 per 1,000 persons, in 1918 it became 17.1, but since then has continued to decline having been as low as 11.6 in 1922 and 10.3 in 1923.

The Possibilities of Further Advance.

When considering the possibilities of enhanced national health it is necessary to distinguish between what is possible as the effect of official action and what must always remain a matter of personal responsibility. If we define Public Health Administration as any action calculated to improve personal or communal health, it has to be considered from the standpoint of (1) the health authorities and their officers, (2) voluntary agencies, (3) educators, including ministers of religion, and (4) the co-operation of the general public; and in fact none of these aspects of the problem can afford to be neglected.

Even if we adopt the more limited definition that the object of Public Health Administration is *to secure the best attainable health of each member of the community, so far as this is or can be secured by the action of local or central authorities concerned with any part of government* the problem is one of greater scope than any central or local governing body has hitherto contemplated.

Thus defined Public Health is not solely a medical problem, though in the present stage of development it is increasingly so. Every local officer of a municipality or other local sanitary authority, from the scavenger to the public analyst, is concerned, and none can claim pride of place. Although now the chief problems of public health are concerned with curative and preventive medicine, as further progress is secured not only will there be further great developments in environmental hygiene on its domestic, social and industrial sides, but physiology including psychology will occupy a more prominent place; and with extensions of knowledge, genetics may advance beyond its present tentative position.

Running through the whole of public health work, which aims at the prevention of the too prevalent human inefficiency and failure, we have a double problem, individual and communal; and our hope of social amelioration lies in continuous study of both these aspects of the problem, in obtaining accurate knowledge of the factors producing inadequacy for the work of life, and in removing these factors.

On its medical side extension of public health work depends firstly on the utilisation of our present physiological and pathological knowledge, and of the chemical and physical sciences which can throw light on the processes of life; and secondly on extension of this knowledge. Much valuable work in this direction is being done by the Medical Research Council, which on the formation of the Ministry of Health was dissociated from the National Health Insurance Commission and placed under the Privy Council, an arrangement which makes its work applicable to Great Britain and more widely, and renders it independent of political influence. The work of this Council is very wide and embraces nearly all branches of investigation. On the general conditions of progress, the following remarks from my official report to the Local Government Board for 1917-18 may be quoted.

Needs of the Future.—The needs for the future may be considered as coming under three chief headings :—

(1) Research into the causation of disease on a much larger scale than has hitherto been attempted.

(2) Extensions of communal action for the prevention and treatment of disease; and more complete training of the medical profession for this work.

(3) Simplification and strengthening of administrative machinery.

Research.—For many years the Local Government Board have undertaken important researches in preventive medicine, so far as the small funds at their disposal have made this practicable. The less limited funds provided for this purpose under the National Insurance Act have already enabled the Medical Research Committee (now Council) to undertake research resulting in considerable advance of our knowledge; and, although during the war, this research work has necessarily been diverted to needs arising out of war conditions these same conditions have led to research work of permanent value. Many problems await the opportunity for further research. It cannot be said that we have advanced far in the knowledge of practicable means for the prevention of catarrhal diseases such as influenza, pneumonia, cerebro-spinal fever and poliomyelitis. The causation and prevention of cancer are still largely unsolved problems. Our knowledge of the underlying problem of immunity is only in its infancy. . . .

But, in addition, research is needed on the part of every medical officer of health and of every medical practitioner. Practice of medicine, whether preventive or curative, in which the practitioner is not engaged also in extending the boundaries of his knowledge, must become steadily less efficient, as the original training of the practitioner recedes. If every medical student were adequately trained in preventive medicine, and if every medical practitioner were given at the State's expense three months' special training in some special branch of medical knowledge once in every third year, the efficiency of the medical service of the community would be greatly increased.

Training.—Not only research, but also a reconstruction of the training of medical students is needed, which will make preventive medicine in its widest sense an integral part of this training, and will ensure that before he begins practice he has definite instruction in the application of the whole of his knowledge to preventive purposes.* The past conception by the public of the relation of medical men to the community—apart from the special case of medical officers of health—has been mistaken. The doctor has been regarded as a help when serious or acute incapacitating illness occurs, and he has but seldom had the opportunity of giving advice in the earlier and more controllable stages of illness. His training has been conducted on the assumption that his chief rôle should be on present lines, with the result that most medical practitioners enter into practice with a too scanty knowledge of hygiene and preventive medicine, and have to learn slowly in belated experience the influence of environment on the health of their patients. The teaching of medicine should be much more largely physiological and hygienic than at present, and such subjects as food values, the hygiene of infancy and childbirth, the physiology of breast feeding, and the influence of environment on the health of their future patients should be the subject of careful training—especially in regard to housing, feeding, clothing, and conditions of work. Were this done, *the ideal condition, in which each medical practitioner becomes a medical officer of health in the range of his own practice*, would approach realisation.

Knowledge of the causation of inefficiency in the community, whether due to disease or to other evils, happily is becoming a more general possession, and every year extensions of public health work

* Action in this direction has recently been stimulated by the General Medical Council.

may be expected, based on this widening view of preventive medicine.

The change is needed. Medicine in the past has furnished many examples of charlatans without exact knowledge, and of specialists who know something almost too well, while ignoring the relationships of their special knowledge to the patient himself. The parallel to this type of specialist in the world of therapeutics is the medical officer of health and sanitary authority who spend money lavishly on an isolation hospital, while neglecting to search out by systematic clinical inquiry or by bacteriological means the "missed" cases which continue to spread infection, and which notifications have not revealed. So also poor law administrators have often been contented to give insufficient or redundant doles, generally unconditional, to the impoverished. Similarly we are learning that while alcoholism is a question of the number of public houses it is also a problem of domestic economy; a problem of monotonous occupation as well as of conviviality; a method of forgetting life under slum conditions as well as a yielding to an insidious habit; and that it needs to be combated from many points as a general problem in preventive social medicine if the attack is to be completely successful. In like manner the medical officer of health is most successful in his work when he convinces all the local authorities in his district—sanitary, educational and parochial—that their respective activities are closely inter-related, and succeeds in obtaining their united aid and that of all available voluntary agencies in removing the evils of municipal and domestic uncleanliness, of overcrowding and defective housing, of insufficient and delayed care of the sick; and when he assists in securing the beneficial results obtainable from the best methods of education and recreation.

While in every branch of social work bearing on the public weal there is need for further research, our present knowledge of the causation of disease suffices for an immediate large extension of its administrative control; and attempts to control disease open up some of the most fertile possibilities of research into further possibilities of control.

To sum up, the principle distinguishing modern medicine is that while not neglecting to apply restorative treatment to the patient, it endeavours to ascertain the causation of his illness and to prevent the continued operation of the causal agents. In the words of the legal maxim, *melius est petere fontes quam rivulos sectari.* A striking illustration of this is embodied in the Reports of the Royal Commission on the Poor Laws, which emphasised the need for searching out and combating the causes of social evil. *This method of approaching social problems, involves the scrapping of some of our older administrative machinery*, just as advance in physical and chemical science necessitates the casting aside of obsolete machinery in the industrial world.

Progress with Imperfect Knowledge.—Although continued advance in public health is dependent chiefly on the utilisation of existent scientific knowledge and on its extension, the history of early sanitary advance shows how much good can be achieved on the basis of imperfect generalisations, such as the one that dirt breeds disease. It was to this hypothesis, which Dr. Southwood Smith, perhaps more than any other medical investigator of the early reform period, advocated and induced Chadwick and his colleagues to apply in practice, that much of our early sanitary administration and its issue in great reduction of disease is owing. To its application may not unreasonably be attributed the disappearance of relapsing and typhus fevers from England, and a remarkable reduction in the amount of typhoid fever. Both typhus and relapsing fevers had ceased to be serious diseases in this country before the specific organisms causing them had been discovered, and before the essential rôle of the louse in inoculating their virus had been ascertained. But improvements in housing were being secured, greater personal and domestic cleanliness was prevailing, and discovered cases of these diseases were being isolated in hospitals; and by these means the links of infection were being interrupted, though doubtless less rapidly than would have occurred had the exact methods of infection been known.

In securing the reduction of disease notwithstanding imperfect knowledge, the increasingly humanitarian outlook of the 18th and of the early part of the 19th Century bore a chief part. John Howard was an early pioneer on these lines. His investigation of prison conditions, described by Edmund Burke as "a voyage of discovery, a circumnavigation of charity," on a plan which "was original, and it was as full of genius as it was of humanity," led to the abolition of typhus from prisons, before a similar success had been achieved outside these. Similarly the work of Percival of Manchester and other reformers led to the introduction of a Bill in 1802, which was the first attempt to diminish child labour. Philanthropic agitation continued and effected the gradual enactment of one Factory Act after another, limiting hours and kinds of work for women and children, and improving industrial conditions generally.

Although imperfect hygienic explanations have been made the basis of successful public health work, explanations without foundation have been the bane of medicine. How much mischief to health has been caused by ascribing disease to *chill*, a conclusion arising from the initial symptom of illness being regarded as its cause. Thackrah of Leeds (1795-1833) early recognised and repudiated this fallacy, asserting of diseases ascribed to the effect of cold or wet

> "nine-tenths . . . wet or cold is no more the cause, even the exciting cause, than Tenterden Steeple of Goodwin Sands."

Hypothesis is necessary for progress, but the constant risk in investigation is of setting out to prove a conviction. As a French scientist has said: "In scientific research be extremely careful for fear you may find exactly what you are looking for."

In every part of his work the public health administrator is surrounded by opportunities of field investigation, particularly in his work for the control of disease. Hence epidemiology is the special science and study of the health officer; and it is by the careful and systematic study of notified cases and the search for unrecognised or concealed cases that he can almost daily add to his armamentarium against disease. It is the officer who loses his keenness and desire to extend the borders of our common knowledge who is especially liable to become a "slacker" in his routine administrative work.

The general moral in work is that we cannot afford to neglect such preventive measures as appear likely to be useful even when our knowledge is imperfect; but that every available research should be pursued, which will convert empirical into rational knowledge. A good instance on this point is seen in Rickets. The importance of hygienic measures and of cod liver oil in the treatment of this serious disease has been long recognised, but the importance of vitamin A and of direct sunshine in its prevention as well as in its cure have now been demonstrated, and this disease will become increasingly rare.

Chapter VI

THE PRINCIPLES OF PUBLIC HEALTH ADMINISTRATION

Already the underlying principles of sound effective public health administration have incidentally been stated in our chiefly historical review of the subject. The same and some further points need to be considered connectedly, before proceeding to describe the present constitution of the Ministry of Health.

We have seen that scattered communities are competent to govern themselves, and that on this is based the ancient supremacy of the Parish as the unit of government; but that increasing human interchanges have necessitated some measure of central or national control over local affairs. Even when central legislation was enacted, as in the Elizabethan Poor Law, the detailed administration nevertheless remained purely local until the year 1834. Matters of Public Health, although dealt with by Poor Law and other local authorities, in the first spasms of reform were controlled by national law and from a central government office; but after a severe revulsion from central control, the balance of central and of local control has varied from decade to decade. In this respect there is much truth in Woodrow Wilson's statement in "An old Master and other Essays":—

"Democratic institutions are never done;

they are like living tissue, always a-making."

Democratic government, whether local or central, i.e. government by elected representatives of the general population, is now almost universal; and it is the duty of everyone to make it successful, in other words to try to combine democracy and efficiency. Though a corrupt motive, both in central and in local government, may often operate, it is literally true, that with large local authorities and in the central Parliament, there is relative safety (from corruption) in numbers. Nor is there need for pessimism as to representative government. As Elihu Root has said in "The Citizen's Part in Government":—

"Pessimism is criminal weakness,"

and study of the worse times that are past is the best cure for pessimism. Until the early part of the 19th century Ministers of the Crown regularly bought the votes of Members of Parliament, and it is not a mere coincidence that at the same period over 200 offences were punishable by death. Occasional scandals and prosecutions for corruption at the present day are evidence rather of the enforcement of a higher standard of public morality than of moral deterioration.

In Great Britain as a rule only the less obvious forms of corruption in public life persist. Among these perhaps the commonest is the giving of representation on an administrative or investigating body to the "interests concerned." The proper place for such persons is in the witness box. Election by the representatives of the public gives the best safeguard against this danger, and even this, owing to the inertia of public opinion does not always suffice.

The case of the National Insurance Act is special. Had it been practicable to nationalise at once all the Friendly Societies, the above rule would apply, minority special representation of the insured being arranged; but in the actual circumstances, especially as the Friendly Societies had large accumulated funds, sectional management preponderantly on behalf of the insured persons unhappily resulted. In practice this has led in many new Societies to completely undemocratic control by large limited liability companies.

Special Consultative Councils have much to be said in their favour as an aid to bureaucratic and to democratic government, these Committees to consist of persons representing interests and of those having special knowledge of the subjects in which administrative work is required. For many years the Home Office and the Board of Education have had such Consultative Committees to advise with the Government Department as to proposed new administrative action before new regulations are enforced.

Similarly the Ministry of Health has formed four such Committees:—

(1) on Medical and Allied Sciences,
(2) on National Health Insurance,
(3) on Local Health Administration,
(4) on General Health Questions.

These Committees can initiate proposals as well as consider proposals submitted to them. They are competent to ensure an adequate hearing for all persons interested professionally or otherwise in proposed action, but decision from the merely interested point of view is avoided by the Committees being advisory only.

With all its drawbacks, government by democracy has proved itself more successful in this country than any preceding form of government, and there is no likelihood of its being superseded.

In government there are three functions: legislative, executive and judicial. In Great Britain the first and second of these centrally are to some extent in the same hands; but both locally and centrally judicial functions as a rule are maintained in complete segregation.

To this salutary rule there are several exceptions. Thus when there is complaint of the professional conduct of a panel doctor, the Ministry of Health appoints a special commission consisting of one barrister and two doctors to report on the facts; the decision as to whether the doctor shall be deprived of his insurance patients rests with the Ministry of Health. The Ministry of Health also acts as a court of appeal when the owner of a house appeals against the decision of the Sanitary Authority ordering the demolition of his insanitary house. Although an appeal lies to the High Court from the Ministry, it is doubtful whether the Ministry should thus act as judge. This function of the Ministry hampers the giving of advice to Local Authorities respecting insanitary property.

The segregation of the judicial part of government is the great safeguard against tyranny either on the part of an individual or of a majority. In England central legislative and executive functions are intimately related, the heads of Departments (Ministers) being directly responsible to Parliament. In the United States members of the Federal Cabinet do not sit in the House of Representatives or Congress. This led Woodrow Wilson, speaking of the Congress, to say: "Deprived of such leadership" (i.e. of the President and his executive) "it becomes a legislative mass meeting instead of a responsible co-operative member of a well organised Government."

There can be no question as to the value of ministerial responsibility to Parliament. The magnificent early efforts of Chadwick and his colleagues were partially wrecked by their excessive zeal, which failed to be tempered by regard for the stage of development of public opinion. Had they been subjected week by week to parliamentary questioning their course would have been impeded; but delayed reform, even when slow and hesitant, is preferable to extreme activity followed ere long by rebellion and stagnation of work. It may be added here that the increase—in connection with "Grants in Aid," etc.—of central control over local public health work makes it increasingly desirable to maintain or even add to the balance of control of the legislature over the permanent executive.

The powers and duties of local health authorities are almost solely executive, the exception being the power to make regulations and by-laws with the approval of the Central Authority concerned. The parish was the original unit of local government, and from this the larger units of local government have been built up. The antiquity of the parish makes it easy to understand with what resentment interference of the Central Government with local affairs has been regarded; but as has already been partially seen the necessities both of poor-law and of public health administration have necessitated large encroachments on local autonomy; in educational administration centralisation has become as marked as in poor-law administration, and much more so than in the region of public health. It is agreed among most local workers that both in regard to education and the poor-law the Central Authority has encroached beyond the limits desirable in the public interest.

What should be the general distribution of central governmental functions? The subject is essentially complex, and a completely satisfactory classification of functions, central and local, probably is impossible. We must be satisfied with an approximation to the best, which will still involve overlapping in places if no hiatus is to be left.

The following Government Departments are concerned with local government, in some degree at least, independently of each other:

The Ministry of Health }
The Board of Control* }
The General Register Office* }
The Home Office,
The Board of Education,
The Ministry of Agriculture and Fisheries,
The Ministry of Labour,
The Ministry of Pensions,

* Officially related to the Ministry of Health.

and most of these central departments are concerned to some extent with problems of health. How is overlapping to be minimised? This subject was ably discussed by a Departmental Committee, of which Lord Haldane was Chairman, in their "Report on the Machinery of Government," which was issued in 1918. This report gives a philosophical presentment of the whole problem, and should be read by all interested in central and local government. The main question is whether the distribution of the functions of Departments shall be (*a*) according to the persons or classes of persons to be dealt with, or (*b*) according to the services to be rendered. Thus there might be a Ministry for children, for insured persons, for paupers, for unemployed. A moment's consideration will show that if each of these Ministries undertook the whole range of requirements for each of these groups, there would arise a gigantic amount of overlapping of work, with deficient application of specialised knowledge, and a reduction of the general standard of government.

The second plan is more logical and more likely to be practical. Thus Education and Health are two great services in general demand for the community, and form fairly natural divisions of ministerial work. These Departments furnish, furthermore, conspicuous examples in which neglect of the principle of classification recommended in the above named report in the past has led to administrative confusion. I refer to the facts that work of medical inspection and treatment of school children was initiated by the Board of Education in 1907-8, and that still more recently administrative disorder was caused by the same Board claiming a share in the hygienic and medical supervision of the præ-school child. (See also p. 133.)

The Ministry of Agriculture and Fisheries furnishes a further example of confused distribution of functions in respect of standards of adulteration of milk, and of control over the distribution of milk from tuberculous cows, with which the Ministry of Health is also concerned.

The most momentous instance of disregard of the rule that government should be arranged according to the chief function involved is the Poor Law or Public Assistance Organisation, both central and local. On the surface it would appear to be otherwise; for the Poor Law deals with the great problem of indigence or destitution. But this view is analogous to the medicine of former days, evidence of which is still visible in our official death returns. Deaths were returned as due to dropsy, ascites, apoplexy, cardiac failure, etc. regardless of the fact that any of these symptoms might be due to any one of several different morbid conditions. Similarly destitution from all causes has been treated as a unity instead of as a complex; and it is only since the issue of the Report of the Royal Commission on the Poor Laws, 1909, that the urgent need for treating the fundamentally differing varieties of destitution by methods suited to their nature and causation has been fully appreciated. In the Central Government vagrancy is a problem for the Home Office rather than for the Ministry of Health; while the vast medical problems of the Poor Law should be administered locally by the large local health authorities. Similarly the local educational work of the Poor Law organisation should be under the Local Education Authorities.

Classification of Government Departments on the lines indicated above is not always practicable; and the three services of National Defence illustrate the fact that on a large scale, and when the persons concerned are adequately segregated in work from the rest of the community, it may be desirable for these services to undertake their own health and medical work. Even in the relation of Education and Health Authorities there is scope for administrative give and take, and inter-departmental conferences as to allied and overlapping work are desirable. Much of the routine work of Education Authorities, e.g. in play and systematic exercises has a medical side, and similarly in the allocation of propaganda and of educational work bearing on health there is need for mutual agreement.

Relation of secretariat to technical officers.—Within each central department of government the relative responsibility of technical and secretarial officials and their relative weight in the counsels of the Parliamentary Head of the Department has been a frequent source of dispute (page 21). Those who read between the lines of Simon's writings, or study what he has written, know full well how important it is that this relationship should be on a satisfactory basis.

In a discussion in the House of Lords during the Great War Lord Sydenham made some remarks revealing what sometimes happens in Government Departments when important problems are under discussion. He said:

> "He believed we had an excellent projectile for the purpose (of destroying a Zeppelin); but owing to the very large number of persons involved in getting anything made for air service we were unable to use the means which science had placed at our disposal. It should be an axiom in Government administration that no one should be permitted to have anything to do with any question on which he could not bring special knowledge to bear. That axiom prevailed in all well managed private businesses. But his own experience, in some Government matters, had been that one had to fight for a necessary improvement through an ascending series of officials, each knowing less than the last, until one reached the deciding authority, who knew nothing at all. This was euphemistically called 'the chain of responsibility.'"

It may be that in the particular instance cited the projectile in question would not do what it was expected to do; and I would add that not only "special knowledge," but also the critical opinion of the trained non-expert is necessary before important administrative action is undertaken. Nevertheless the quotation aptly states the gradual "snowing under" of expert advice which not infrequently occurs probably in all Government Departments.

This is not to claim that the final decision should rest with the expert adviser. Considerations of practicability or expediency or public policy must necessarily enter into any proposal of reform. What is required to secure satisfaction and efficiency is that the technical adviser, medical or other, shall always be present at the Ministerial Conference at which important administrative measures on which he has advised, or ought to have been called upon to advise, are considered. Instead of this the Minister not infrequently knows of his skilled technical adviser's views only through a summarised minute written by the Minister's private or departmental secretary, or through a verbal statement of these views by his secretary; and the Minister may decide important questions in the feeble and possibly distorted light of imperfect or biased knowledge, possibly founded on expediency or timidity, or on personal prejudice.

Democratic government has not a fair chance of success unless the Minister representing the public determines to refuse to be a mere echo of his secretarial officials, or if he does not consider in open conference the contentions of his technical as well as of his secretarial advisers.

What are the respective duties of the Central and the Local Public Health Administration?

The two branches of administration are in indissoluble partnership, and the shifting problem as to the best means for securing the maximum benefit to the community from their joint administration is one of great interest and importance.

A comparison of the problem with that of the successful organisation in the human body of the control of the nervous system over the bodily functions is useful. There are three levels of nervous activity. The brain cells control thought and volition; intermediate cells govern movements which are fairly complicated, as those of walking; while peripheral nervous elements direct the simplest movements in life. Thus by the application of what has been called a *doctrine of levels*, economy and efficiency of effort is secured in every part of the human system.

(*a*) The first condition of such efficiency in Public Health is the application for routine public health administration of the absolutely sound recommendation made by the Royal Sanitary Commission of 1869:

> "All powers requisite for the health of town and country should in every place be possessed by one responsible local authority . . . so that no area should be without such an authority, or have more than one."

(*b*) The second condition is so to balance central and local control as to secure maximum efficiency with the minimum amount of interference with local initiative.

Much of the failure to secure these two conditions of good government has arisen from the ineptitude and ignorance of many of our legislators. For these—and for the more responsible officials—a compulsory period of training or actual experience in local administration before they become eligible for legislative work, would greatly increase the efficiency of the public service.

(*c*) It would further conduce greatly to the efficiency of central administration and its satisfactory adjustment to local needs, were it practicable to arrange for opportunities to serve for a period with local authorities to be given to secretaries of Departments before they take on their secretarial duties. One of the chief difficulties in central administration is the lack of knowledge on the part of central administrators of local administration; and the provision of interchange between central and local departments would materially enhance the efficiency of national service.

(*d*) A fourth condition is that, as indicated in the physiological analogy suggested above, the central health authority should concern itself with major matters and should avoid pernickity checking of the detailed work of local authorities, always subject to their fulfilling a minimum standard in the various branches of public health administration. It would not be difficult to formulate such a *series of standards* for different grades of sanitary authorities, conformity with which on the certificate of the responsible chief officials of the authority would minimise detailed inspection from the central authority, and the making of over-elaborate periodical returns in respect of grant-aided activities.

(*e*) The physiological illustration, when applied to modern conditions, indicates a necessary limitation of the sound rule stated by the Royal Commission in 1869. At that time the main problems were local and limited in scope—scavenging, water supplies, fever hospitals, sewerage, etc. The rapid growth of population and the overflow of population from urban to rural areas have created novel problems, necessitating larger units of government for special purposes. The relation of the county council to the constituent sanitary areas in a county illustrates this. For certain purposes this does not suffice. Thus schemes of water supply on a large scale may necessitate combined action on behalf of several towns and of a large county area. The West Riding Rivers Pollution Board furnishes a further example of administrative action overlapping many sanitary areas. A county and a county borough area contiguous to each other may form very uneconomical units for the provision of hospital accommodation; and machinery for compulsory joint action is needed. The Metropolitan Asylums Board is a good illustration of the value of pooling provision of hospitals for fever, for smallpox, for tuberculosis, and for mental deficiency, etc. for the entire metropolis. The question as to the method of appointment of such joint bodies needs careful consideration.

Chapter VII

THE MINISTRY OF HEALTH

THE general considerations advanced in the preceding chapter, following on the history of the development of public health work sketched in earlier chapters, should now enable us to formulate the proper functions of the Ministry of Health, as developed from those of its predecessor, the Local Government Board, with added functions from other Government Departments.

The Local Government Board had as its chief functions :—

(1) The control of relief of the poor.

(2) The powers previously in the hands of the Privy Council as to public vaccination.

(3) Powers as to the registration of marriages, births and deaths.

(4) Supervision with some control of the local administration of the laws relating to the public health.

(5) Similar supervision and control in relation to local government.

(6) Returns as to taxation.

And the chief means employed in carrying out the special public health part of this work were, and under the Ministry of Health continue to be, as follows :—

(1) Supervision of the work of local authorities,

and efforts to co-ordinate the work of different local authorities so as to secure the maximum of efficiency.

(2) Inspection of local work by skilled medical officers, who while (*a*) thus obtaining evidence of failure or defect of work, especially (*b*) in connection with work for which the Ministry give grants in aid, should be more concerned with (*c*) the giving of helpful counsel to local officers, and (*d*) putting these officers in touch with recent advances in public health knowledge or work that may advantageously be utilised.

(3) The giving of grants in aid of local work.

So far as Public Health is concerned, the Local Government Board was hampered throughout its forty-eight years' existence by its poor law duties and traditions; and the old ideals of poor law administration to the last prevailed in its counsels, though steadily decreasing in influence. The extent to which local and central public health administration succeeded notwithstanding this heavy handicap can be gathered from the contents of pages 64 to 71.

The duties of the Ministry of Health are briefly defined in the Ministry of Health Act, 1919. In the first clause it is proposed to appoint a Minister of Health "for the purpose of promoting the health of the people throughout England and Wales, and for the purpose of the exercise of the powers transferred or conferred by this Act."

The general powers and duties of the Minister in relation to health are defined in the second clause as follows:—

to take all such steps as may be desirable to secure the preparation, effective carrying out and co-ordination of measures conducive to the health of the people, including measures for the prevention and cure of diseases, the avoidance of fraud in connection with alleged remedies therefor, the treatment of physical and mental defects, the treatment and care of the blind, the initiation and direction of research, the collection, preparation, publication, and dissemination of information and statistics relating thereto, and the training of persons for health services.

By clause 3 important duties are transferred to the Minister of Health :—

(*a*) all the powers and duties of the Local Government Board ;

(*b*) all the powers and duties of the Insurance Commissioners and the Welsh Insurance Commissioners ;

(*c*) all the powers of the Board of Education with respect to attending to the health of expectant mothers and nursing mothers and of children who have not attained the age of five years and are not in attendance at schools recognised by the Board of Education ;

(*d*) all the powers and duties of the Board of Education with respect to the medical inspection and treatment of children and young persons under paragraph (*b*) of subsection (1) of section thirteen of the Education (Administrative Provisions) Act, 1907, as amended and extended by the Education Act, 1918: Provided that, for the purpose of facilitating the effective exercise and performance of these powers and duties, the Minister may make arrangements with the Board of Education respecting the submission and approval of schemes of local education authorities and the payment of grants to local education authorities, so far as such schemes and payment relate to or are in respect of medical inspection and treatment; and the powers and duties of the Minister may under any such arrangements be exercised and performed by the Board on his behalf and with his authority under such conditions as he may think fit;

(*e*) all the powers of the Privy Council and of the Lord President of the Council under the Midwives Acts, 1902 and 1918;

(*f*) such powers of supervising the administration of Part I. of the Children Act, 1908 (which relates to infant life protection), as have heretofore been exercised by the Secretary of State:

Provided that—

A the power conferred on the Insurance Commissioners by the proviso to subsection (2) of section sixteen of the National Insurance Act, 1911, of retaining and applying for the purposes of research such sums as are therein mentioned shall not be transferred to the Minister, but the duties heretofore performed by the Medical Research Committee shall after the date of the commencement of this Act be carried on by or under the direction of a Committee of the Privy Council appointed by His Majesty for that purpose, and any property held for the purposes of the former Committee shall after that date be transferred to and vested in such persons as the body by whom such duties as aforesaid are carried on may appoint, and be held by them for the purposes of that body; and

(ii) in such matters of a judicial nature under the National Insurance (Health) Acts, 1911 to 1918, as may be prescribed under those Acts, the powers and duties of the Insurance Commissioners and the Welsh Insurance Commissioners by this Act transferred to the Minister shall be exercised by the Minister through a special body or special bodies of persons constituted in such manner as may be so prescribed.

B It shall be lawful for His Majesty from time to time by Order in Council to transfer to the Minister—

(*a*) all or any of the powers and duties of the Minister of Pensions with respect to the health of disabled officers and men after they have left the service;

(*b*) all or any of the powers and duties of the Secretary of State under the enactments relating to lunacy and mental deficiency;

(*c*) any other powers and duties in England and Wales of any Government department which appear to His Majesty to relate to matters affecting or incidental to the health of the people.

C It shall be lawful for His Majesty from time to time by Order in Council to transfer from the Minister to any other Government department any of the powers and duties of the Minister, whether relating to the relief of the poor or otherwise, which appear to His Majesty not to relate to matters affecting or incidental to the health of the people.

And it is hereby declared that it is the intention of this Act that, in the event of provision being made by Act of Parliament passed in the present or in any future session for the revision of the law relating to the relief of the poor and the distribution amongst other authorities of the powers exercisable by boards of guardians, there shall be transferred from the Minister to other Government departments such of the powers and duties under the enactments relating to the relief of the poor then vested in the Minister (not being powers or duties relating or incidental to the health of the people) as appear to His Majesty to be such as could be more conveniently exercised and performed by such other departments.

(4) His Majesty may by Order in Council make such incidental, consequential, and supplemental provisions as may be necessary or expedient for

the purpose of giving full effect to any transfer of powers or duties by or under this section, including provisions for the transfer of any property, rights, and liabilities held, enjoyed, or incurred by any Government department in connection with any powers or duties transferred, and may make such adaptations in the enactments relating to such powers or duties as may be necessary to make exercisable by the Minister and his officers or by such other Government department and their officers, as the case may be, the powers and duties so transferred.

(5) In connection with the transfer of powers and duties to or from the Minister by or under this Act, the provisions set out in the First Schedule to this Act shall have effect.

The fourth and fifth clauses run as follows:—

4.—(1) It shall be lawful for His Majesty by Order in Council to establish consultative councils in England and Wales for giving, in accordance with the provisions of the Order, advice and assistance to the Minister in connection with such matters affecting or incidental to the health of the people as may be referred to in such Order.

(2) Every such council shall include women as well as men, and shall consist of persons having practical experience of the matters referred to the council.

5.—The Minister shall, subject to the provisions of this Act, appoint such officers as he may think fit to constitute a Board of Health in Wales through whom he may exercise and perform in Wales in such manner as he may think fit any of his powers and duties; the Board and any officer who is a member thereof shall act under the directions, and comply with the instructions, of the Minister.

It will be observed that in the formation of the Ministry of Health provision was made for assembling under the Ministry the duties hitherto discharged by the Local Government Board and those of the National (Health) Insurance Commission. This at once removed one of the greatest difficulties to efficient central health work, which the National Insurance Act had created. When this Act was passed unfortunately both the Local Government Board and the Board of Education were already actively engaged in medical and hygienic work, in considerable measure for the same persons. The addition of the Insurance Medical work, in a third compartment, multiplied confusion and seriously impeded satisfactory work. Incidentally it also postponed the poor-law medical reform, in favour of which the Royal Commission on the Poor Laws had reported, and so a momentous opportunity for unifying the medical work of government was allowed to slip.

In the second place the Ministry of Health Act transferred to the new Ministry the powers and duties of the Board of Education with respect to præ-school children and to school children; but subject to the important proviso in respect of school children, quoted on page 99. In fact there is still in many localities and there continues in the Board of Education and the Ministry of Health a large measure of administrative separation between the public health and the educational medical services, notwithstanding the fact that a partial liaison is established centrally by the fact that there is one chief medical officer for both Departments. It is however, an exaggeration to state (*Public Health*, Nov., 1924) that "the separation of the medical work of the Board of Education from the Ministry of Health is just as complete as ever, and any alleged unification in that direction is merely make believe."

The anomaly of present arrangements is especially marked in regard to medical institutions for children of school age. Thus the supervision of institutions for orthopædic cases rests with the Board of Education; for persons below and over school age, who may be treated in the same institution as school children, inspection devolves upon the Ministry of Health; and similar anomalies may arise in local administration.

Local amalgamation of the medical work for children of school age and at lower ages is even more important than its central unification. This work, like central supervision, has an educational as well as a medical side; and no action should be taken which will decrease the active interest of the local Education Committee, and still more of the school teacher, in the detailed work of medical inspection and treatment of school children. In most educational areas joint action is being successfully achieved by combined meetings of education and public health committees, and by bringing the teachers and school attendance officers into conference and consultation with the school medical officer. As school medical inspection becomes increasingly preventive and less palliative and curative in its scope, the necessity for active daily partnership between hygienic and scholastic workers in every area will increase.

3rd. The transfer of the powers of the Privy Council under the Midwives Acts to the Ministry of Health brought the Central Midwives Board and the Local Supervising Authorities (County Councils and County Borough Councils) into their due relationship to the Ministry. The Central Midwives Board is a statutory body, having the duty of keeping a roll of qualified midwives, and with disciplinary powers, enabling it to suspend from practice or strike off the roll midwives guilty of *mala praxis*.

4th. The central control of Part I of the Children Act relating to Infant Protection was transferred from the Home Office to the Ministry of Health. The local supervision of children under seven years of age in the provinces is still, however, in the hands of Boards of Guardians, instead of being the work of the public health authority which is engaged in other parts of infant and child welfare work; and for this important reform we must await further legislation.

5th. As already indicated, the transfer of the work of the Medical Research Committee to the department of the Privy Council enables it to function for both England and Scotland, and gives a prospect of steady continuity to this extremely important branch of public health work.

6th. It will be noted that the Ministry of Health is empowered but not required to take over certain duties of the Home Office as to lunacy and of the Ministry of Pensions as to ex-service men.

The Board of Control, which forms the Central Authority for lunatics and mental defectives, is the legal successor of the Lunacy Commission, which was appointed in 1845 as a permanent Government Commission. The Lunacy Commissioners were half of them legal and half of them medical and their main duty was the visitation of institutions in which insane persons were detained; generally they exercised control over lunacy administration. The Commissioners were appointed by the Lord Chancellor.

Under the Mental Deficiency Act, 1913, the Lunacy Commission was merged in the Board of Control, and the powers of the Board were considerably enlarged. The Act provides that the Board shall consist of not more than fifteen Commissioners, of whom not more than twelve shall be paid; and that of the paid Commissioners four shall be legal and four medical. It also enacts that at least one of the paid and one of the unpaid Commissioners shall be a woman. The legal members are appointed by the Lord Chancellor and the Chairman and the other members by the Minister of Health.

The duties of the Board of Control now comprise the supervision of mental defectives as well as the supervision of the insane. To a very large extent the Board of Control is an independent body, but its estimates are submitted to Parliament by the Minister of Health which gives the Minister general jurisdiction. On certain financial matters, such as the sanctioning of loans, the approving of contracts both in regard to lunacy and mental deficiency, the express sanction of the Minister is required.

By the Ministry of Health (Lunacy and Mental Deficiency, Transfer of Powers) Order, 1920 (S.R.O. 809), most of the powers of the Secretary of State in regard to lunacy and mental deficiency were transferred to the Minister of Health.

The Transfer of Powers Order did not affect the powers of the Board of Education. Defective children of school age still remain under the jurisdiction of the local education authorities unless they are notified to the mental deficiency authority as being incapable by reason of mental defect of receiving benefit in a Special school or that they cannot be instructed in a Special school without detriment to the interests of the other children.

The number of places in Special schools is not nearly sufficient to accommodate the number of defective school children.

The expenditure of local authorities (county councils and county borough councils or joint committees of such councils) in carrying out their duties in regard to cases of mental deficiency is partly covered by Exchequer grants. The medical officer of health acts as the "certifying officer" under the service.

The terms of the Ministry of Health Act do not provide for the transfer from the Home Office of the central control over occupational diseases and over factory hygiene. The Home Office also still controls the provision of burial grounds, and the control of inebriates. Local authorities have certain duties as to cleanliness and drainage of factories, and as to the provision of fire escapes, which centrally come under the Home Office.

The Home Office is the Department charged with the administration of the Dangerous Drugs Acts, which aim at the prevention of addiction to drugs. These Acts give effect to the Opium Convention of 1912 by imposing stringent restrictions on the importation, exportation, and distribution of opium, morphia, cocaine and heroin. Important obligations devolve upon doctors and pharmacists in prescribing and dispensing these drugs. Records of their purchase and supply must be kept and be open to inspection. By arrangement between the Home Office and the Ministry of Health the records kept by doctors and hospitals are carried out by the Regional Medical Staff of the Ministry.

That it is impracticable to separate completely the health functions and other duties of central administration may be inferred from the continuing oversight of the Ministry of Health over many branches of local administration. In fact the Ministry of Health remains a Local Government Board from which a few non-hygienic duties have been relegated to the Home Office and other Departments of Government. These are registration and elections, transferred to the Home Office, public libraries and museums to the Board of Education, and some powers over gas undertakings to the Board of Trade.

The additional powers given to the Ministry of Health have been already enumerated. To these may be added the more stringent and extensive powers given under recent Housing and Town Planning Acts.

Other functions of the Ministry, only indirectly related to health are concerned with

Private Bill legislation as to finance,
Questions of valuation and local taxation,
Schemes to relieve unemployment,
Audit of local accounts,
Old age pensions (final appeals on).

As showing the magnitude of the expenditure of local authorities with which the Ministry of Health is concerned the following figures are taken from the Ministry's Fifth Annual Report for 1923-24.

Financial Position of Local Authorities in 1921-22 (including all Sanitary Authorities, County Councils, Boards of Guardians and Water Boards).

	£
Expenditure defrayed otherwise than out of loans ..	365,025,768
Expenditure defrayed out of loans	128,729,894
Receipts from—	
Rates	170,871,876
Government grants	76,663,078
Other sources, not being loans (e.g. tramways, electric light works, etc.)	126,932,884
Outstanding external loan debt	768,566,752

Financial Central Control.—The control of the Ministry of Health, as in the past of the Local Government Board, over the granting of Loans gives it an important voice in large-scaled local expenditure. It imposes the conditions that (1) the loan applied for is for works of a more or less permanent character, (2) that the loan is for a limited amount, (3) that the payment of interest and repayment of the loan is chargeable against the rates or revenue account, (4) that the period of repayment is within a fixed period. This varies from ten to thirty years; exceptionally it may extend to sixty or even eighty years.

The most drastic control over current expenditure of local authorities and over the manner of its expenditure, is in connection with the *Grants in Aid* given to them by the central government. These are 50 per cent. of approved local expenditure on

Maternity and Child Welfare work and on Tuberculosis work;

and 75 per cent. of approved local expenditure on

Venereal Disease schemes (see pages 209, 222, 233).

The total amount of such grants exceeded 74 millions sterling in the financial year 1922-23. Of this amount

£1,936,564 was paid to local authorities	for tuberculosis services.
£882,556 „ „ „ „ „	in connection with their maternity & child welfare schemes.
£407,277 „ „ „ „ „	for venereal disease services.
£389,174 „ „ „ „ „	for salaries of sanitary officers.
£10,323 „ „ „ „ „	for vaccination.
£45,464 „ „ „ „ „	port sanitary service.
£83,470 was distributed to voluntary agencies and local authorities	for work for the blind.

These amounts may be compared with Exchequer Grants in the same year of £42,867,563 for Education, of £1,431,671 for Lunatics and Mental Defectives, of £4,733,285 for Housing, of £9,413,254 for the Police, and of £1,180,178 for Relief of the Poor, besides £2,437,428 unallocated and other sums.

The relative magnitude of total local rates which these grants supplement is seen in the following figures extracted from the 5th Report of the Ministry of Health. They give the percentages of the amount of total local rates received in the year 1921-22, applied in meeting expenditure on each of the principal groups of local services.

		Per cent. of total rates.
Education (including public libraries)		19.4
Highways and bridges		17.7
Health :—		
(1) Sewers, water supply, hospitals, vaccination, salaries of health officers, etc. etc.	17.7	
(2) Maternity and child welfare, tuberculosis, venereal diseases	0.9	
(3) Lunacy and mental deficiency ..	3.8	
		22.4
Housing and town planning..		0.6
Relief of the poor		18.9
Administration of justice, police, fire brigades ..		7.7
Other services or services not allocated		13.3
Total		100.0

The *Grant in Aid system* in aid of local rates has much to be said for it and against it. The ability of local authorities to carry out necessary public health work varies greatly with local social conditions, and grants in aid tend to diminish anomalies in the incidence of local expenditure. The promise of a fifty-fifty grant for expenditure on tuberculosis and child welfare schemes or of a seventy-five—twenty-five grant on venereal disease schemes has proved a distinct incitement to local authorities to undertake these special branches of work and to improve them when begun. Grants in aid are also given to foster police efficiency, they form a large part of educational and of poor law expenditure, they are given in half-payment of the salaries of many health officers, and more recently they have been given for the new developments of public health work mentioned above. The poor law grant is not dependent on efficiency of work; but on the public health side the more recent grants have been effective in securing rapid increase in important public health services, and their abolition without substitution of some other form of central grant which like the present grants would stimulate local work, would be a calamity. However ingrained in the public mind is the desire for local control of local affairs, Exchequer Grants in some form or other are likely to continue and to increase, thus making local authorities and the central government partners and joint directors in the local undertakings to which both have contributed funds.

This co-partnership can be made to work efficiently subject to certain general conditions which hitherto have not been adequately secured.

1st. No grants should be given except to local authorities of a magnitude which will furnish some guarantee of efficient and satisfactory administration, and safeguard in large measure against over-officering or incompetent officering. This involves the revision of local governmental areas advocated in Chapter IV.

2nd. The public health work to which the funds of dual source are devoted should be regulated by general conditions laid down by the Ministry of Health after adequate consultation with and approval by the local authorities about to receive central contributions. Arrangements might be made for local authorities to give this approval in some collective capacity.

3rd. No official grants in aid should be given to any local voluntary association, except through the medium of the local county council or county borough council in whose area the association works; and the county council should be utilised to a much greater extent than at present in supervising the grant-earning work of the sanitary authorities within the county area.

4th. Subject to fulfilment of the above conditions, central authorities might curtail detailed systematic inspection and inquiry respecting the local administration of the grants, which may easily become pernickity. There must, of course, be financial check on expenditure; but subject to special exceptions, comparative statistics should give this without inquiries into minute details. The fulfilment of this fourth suggestion would give increased elasticity and spontaneity to local work, and stimulate originality and progress in both the educational and public health spheres of work.

Details of some of the grant-earning services of local authorities are given in subsequent chapters.

Chapter VIII

OTHER CENTRAL HEALTH AUTHORITIES:

A. The Factory Department of the Home Office

The Ministry of Health as established by the Ministry of Health Act, 1919, represents an important advance in central unification of the health services of the State. The domiciliary medical treatment of one-third of the total population, previously regulated in separate departments by the National Health Insurance Commissioners and the Welsh Insurance Commissioners, was transferred with the total insurance work of these Commissions to the Local Government Board, the chief Central Department of Health for England and Wales, and they were re-named the Ministry of Health. Prior to this event, the public health division of Local Government Board and local sanitary authorities had, especially in regard to children, extended their activities on the treatment side of disease-prevention beyond the acute and chronic infections. The new fusion, once for all stamped with the approval of the legislature the two fundamentally important conceptions that the State, on a much wider scale, is vitally concerned in securing for the community medical treatment of all kinds of illness; and that treatment and prevention are inseparably bound together, if effort in either direction is to command success.

The Ministry of Health Act furthermore contemplated the early transference of the powers and duties of the Board of Education as to medical inspection and treatment of school children to the new Ministry. These duties are of such an extent and so important to the welfare of the community as to deserve the designation of a separate Ministry of Health.

There is no mention of the important health duties of the Home Office under the Factory Acts in the Ministry of Health Act, and evidently complete if any transfer of these was not contemplated; and yet there inheres in this Department of State a vast responsibility in health matters which justifies its description—as has recently been done—by Lieut.-Col. F. E. Fremantle, M.D., M.P., as a third Ministry of Health.

Transfers from the Home Office.—Notwithstanding the absence of definite provision to this effect, some minor transfers have been effected from the Home Office. The exact and limited extent of these transfers is seen in the following extract from a circular issued by the Ministry of Health in October, 1921 (Circ. 235).

This circular forwards for the information of the Local Authority, copies of the Ministry of Health (Factories and Workshops Transfer of Powers) Order, 1921, made under the Ministry of Health Act by which the powers and duties of the Secretary of State, under the undermentioned Sections of the Factory and Workshop Act, 1901, are transferred to the Minister of Health, namely :—

Sec. 61.—Prohibition of employment of women after childbirth.

Sec. 97-100.—Provisions relating to bakehouses.

Sec. 109.—Making of wearing apparel where there is scarlet fever or smallpox.

Sec. 110.—Prohibition of Homework where there is infectious disease.

Prohibition of Employment of Women after Childbirth.

Section 61 of the Act provides that the occupier of a factory or workshop shall not knowingly allow a woman or girl to be employed therein within four weeks after she has given birth to a child. This Section is extended to laundries by Section 103 of the Act.

The Minister trusts that local authorities administering Maternity and Child Welfare Schemes will assist occupiers of factories, workshops, and laundries in observing the provisions of this Section, so far as they are in a position to do so. He would be glad if all local authorities would in the future communicate with this Department on any points which may arise under this Section.

Bakehouses.

It seems to the Minister that the enforcement of the provisions relating to bakehouses can better be undertaken locally than centrally, especially as the work is of the same character as that at present performed by the sanitary staff of local authorities in relation to retail bakehouses under Section 102 of the Act of 1901.

The actual amount of additional work involved will be very small, as it is believed that the number of wholesale bakehouses in England and Wales is less than two thousand.

In addition to their duties in relation to retail bakehouses under Section 102, local authorities are also charged with the certification of underground bakehouses under Section 101. Under Section 98 the Authority have concurrent powers with the Factory Inspector to undertake a prosecution in the case of a bakehouse which is unsuitable on sanitary grounds. The Minister understands that the power of prosecution under this Section has in the past been mainly exercised by the Factory Inspector, but he suggests that in future it should be wholly exercised by the local authority. Local Authorities have no specific powers of enforcement in regard to Sections 97, 99 and 100, but it is suggested that where an offence is committed under any of these Sections, and the defect is not remedied at the suggestion of the authority, proceedings could usually be undertaken under the general terms of Section 98. In any case, where this cannot be done, the Minister would be glad if the facts were referred to him.

Reference may also be made to Section 125 under which the local authority and their officers have all necessary powers of entry, inspection, etc.

Homework in Infected Premises.

The powers and duties of local authorities under Sections 109 and 110, relating to homework in premises where there is infectious disease are not affected by the transfer to the Minister of jurisdiction in regard to these Sections, and there is no alteration of the classes of work to which the Sections have hitherto applied.

The Minister considers it desirable, however, to draw the attention of the local authorities to the provisions of subsection 5 of Section 110 under which the Section may be applied by special order of the Secretary of State (now the Minister of Health) to other classes of work besides those specified in the subsection, and to Part II of the Homework Order of the 23rd May, 1907, which applied the subsection to various classes of work in addition to those specified therein. (*End of Extract.*)

* * *

The vast extent of the sanitary regulations as to Factories and Workshops now under the centralised control of the Factory Department of the Home Office may be seen by reference to the Factory Acts and to the important regulations made under them. The extent to which the Factory Department of the Home Office regulates local industrial health matters can be judged from a persual of the "Factory and Workshop Orders" (1924 edition). Among these orders the following may be selected for mention :—

(1) Order (1902) modifying the proportion of cubic feet of space in workshops used as sleeping places.

(2) Order (1903) modifying the proportion of cubic feet of space to be provided in certain bake-houses.

(3) Order (1903) as to number of sanitary conveniences to be provided in factories.

(4) Various Orders as to Hours and Holidays, as to Meal Times, as to Overtime, as to Night work.

(5) Orders applying the application of Sub-

section 4 of Section 73 of the Factory and Workshop Act, 1901, for the notification to H.M. Chief Inspector of Factories, Whitehall, S.W., of cases of lead or phosphorus poisoning, of anthrax, etc., arising from factory work, also to cases of toxic jaundice (1915), and to epitheliomatous and chronic ulceration (1919).

(6) Order (1898) prohibiting the taking of meals in certain places.

(7) Order as to Humid Textile Factories, 1892.

(8) Orders as to Home Work.

(9) Regulations for Dangerous Trades.

a Manufacture of felt hats, where any inflammable solvent is used (1902).
b File-cutting by hand (1903).
c Manufacture of electric accumulators (1903).
d Handling, etc., of goods in docks, quays, etc.
e Sorting of wool, goat-hair and camel-hair.
f Spinning and weaving of flax and tow.
g Manufacture of paints and colours.
h The use of horsehair.
i The casting of brass.
j The vitreous enamelling of metal or glass.
k Electrical plants, tinning of metal-ware, grinding of metals, lead smelting, bronzing, the manufacture of pottery, of lead compounds, of celluloid, the handling of hides and skins, and many others.

Factory hygiene historically in some measure anticipated general hygiene; and official control over it has always been almost completely divorced from local health authorities. Medical considerations enter largely into the questions concerned in the hygienic control of the 140,000 factories and 145,000 workshops in Great Britain; and yet both centrally and locally the association of industrial hygiene with the chief public health services (the Ministry of Health and local public health authorities) is so slight as to be nearly negligible. On questions of dust and of industrial poisoning and infections the medical officer of health and sanitary inspector have no right of entry into factories, and sanitary authorities and local insurance committees must be contented with arranging for the treatment of the cases of phthisis, of anthrax, of lead poisoning which originate in badly controlled factory life. It is not suggested that the four medical inspectors and the 200 lay district inspectors of the Factory Department of the Home Office have not done magnificent work in diminishing dust, and in safeguarding workers against impure air, against accident, and against overwork. Furthermore, the fact that these inspectors act for large areas and are not limited to the region of one county borough or county council has ensured freedom from local pressure against reform and has enabled inspectors to gain experience in needed devices for preventing danger from accident, or dust, which could not always be expected from locally appointed officers. Nevertheless, the divorce between central and local health administration, especially on its medical side, is unfortunate and the time has arrived when it should be revised. It is true that there is a local medical link in the Certifying Factory Surgeon, whose fourfold duties are stated by Sir T. M. Legge, C.B.E., the Senior Medical Inspector of the Home

Office (*Journ. Roy. Sanitary Inst.*, Nov., 1924) to be:—

(1) Examination of young persons under 16 years of age within seven days of their employment in a factory;

(2) Investigation of notified industrial diseases and gassing cases;

(3) Periodical medical examination of workers in dangerous trades under Regulations; and

(4) Granting certificates entitling to compensation under the Workmen's Compensation Act.

The Factory Surgeon is appointed by the Home Office, and is a well qualified medical man engaged also in private practice. He is seldom the medical officer of health. It is desirable that he should be more closely linked up with the school medical officer, if not actually the same officer, and should be possessed of the past medical history of the young person examined by him as to fitness for factory employment.

It is also desirable that the local medical officer of health should be made acquainted with the Certifying Surgeon's inquiries even when it cannot be arranged for the medical officer of health to undertake these inquiries. In some instances, at least, the diseases notified by local medical practitioners to the Factory Department in London also occur outside factories; and factory and extra-factory investigation should be pursued side by side.

The first appointment of medical officer of health, that of Liverpool, was made in 1847, while the first Certifying Factory Surgeon was appointed under the Factory Act of 1844. At that time his sole duty was that of certifying the age of the young person entering the factory, thus safeguarding against premature industrial employment, and determining fitness for work in a factory. The appointment was one in personal hygiene, rather than in environmental hygiene to which the duties of the medical officer of health in later years were first chiefly directed. The certifying factory surgeon thus was the forerunner of the school doctor. Similarly, with exceptions in a number of provincial towns, the school medical officer preceded the doctor attached to the child welfare centre. The stages were illogical and topsy-turvy, but needs were met as they were realised; and the State is gradually advancing to a system of increasingly complete hygienic and medical provision for the community, beginning with the pregnant mother, becoming fairly complete for the infant, less complete for the child aged 1-5 years, still very incomplete for the scholar in elementary and secondary schools, rudimentary for the young person entering employment, and in later life supplied—though in practice only when sickness occurs—for one-third of the general population from 16 years old onward under the National Insurance Act.

Is there not need for devolution of the medical functions of the Factory Department of the Home Office in regard to examination of young persons beginning work in factories, and in regard to investigation of cases of industrial poisoning and infection, if not also for the details of local factory hygiene? I think there is; and that better work would be done if this were arranged, the inspectors, medical and non-medical, of the Home Office retaining their supervisory and consultative functions, while they would not be overloaded with their present executive detail, nor overwhelmed with the multitude of local inspections requiring to be made. Some risk of temporary reduction of efficiency would be incurred; but the time for devolution is overdue; and continuance of the main features of central supervision are quite consistent with this.

As regards central supervision of factory hygiene, the views of the Committee on the Machinery of Government may be quoted at this point:—

> "26. We are only in a position to suggest that in existing circumstances certain services do not seem to us to be proper for inclusion in the sphere of the Ministry of Health, at any rate at the outset.
>
> "27. We may mention, as examples, the duties of the Home Office in safeguarding the health of industrial workers, and the new developments of work in the same field which have taken place under the supervision of the Ministry of Munitions; the work of the Board of Trade in safeguarding the health of the Mercantile Marine under the Merchant Shipping Acts; and the duties of the Board of Agriculture and Fisheries in regard to the inspection of milk and food. . . . These duties of the Home Office seem to us to be most appropriate to the Department charged with the general supervision of industrial conditions. The inspection of milk and food is a matter which seems to us necessarily to involve the consideration of the different points of view

at present represented by the Board of Agriculture and the Local Government Board, and it will probably be necessary for a Ministry of Health to continue to deal with these matters in conjunction with the Board of Agriculture. Similar provision should also be made for regular consultation between the Ministry of Health and the Board of Trade on questions affecting the health of the Mercantile Marine.

"28. In other cases it is scarcely open to doubt that the promotion of physical well-being is a subordinate, although an indispensable element, in a service primarily devoted to other ends. It would not, for example, be suggested that a Ministry of Health should take over the medical services of the Ministries of Defence (Admiralty, War Office and Air Ministry), or the organisation established by the Ministry of National Service, which has for its primary object the recruiting of the Army; or the Medical Department by means of which the Postmaster-General attends to the health of his employees.

"29. But to say that these subordinate health services should remain separate from the main services of the same kind for which the Ministry of Health would be responsible is not to imply that there should be any want of communication between that Ministry and the Departments concerned with health administration as a subdivision of their main business. On the contrary, we suggest that it should be a most important function of the Ministry of Health to arrange for frequent consultation, and to secure full co-operation in health matters, between its officers, both professional and administrative, and the officers of other Departments engaged in such work as we have mentioned. There is perhaps no province of affairs in which the exchange of suggestions and criticism is more necessary to progress, or productive of more certain results."

I have quoted this statement in full, because it states the general case for retention of certain health functions in charge of central departments other than the Ministry of Health. With the exception of the problems of factory hygiene, these health functions of the Board of Agriculture, of the Board of Trade, and of the Home Office may be regarded as ancillary to other closely related functions; and the difficulty of more than one central government department being concerned in health matters may be regarded as a less evil than separation for instance of problems of safe machinery from those of dusty industrial operations.

There is much to be said on both sides as regards central supervision of factory hygiene. Theoretically it ought to belong to the Ministry of Health with other branches of supervision of local health functions.

The following are the special sub-departments of medical work in the Ministry of Health:—

MEDICAL DEPARTMENT OF THE MINISTRY OF HEALTH.

Chief Medical Officer.

(1) *General Health and Epidemiology.*

One Senior Medical Officer, and 14 Medical Officers.

(2) *Maternity and Child Welfare.*
One Senior Medical Officer, 4 Medical Officers, 5 Nurse Inspectors.

(3) *Tuberculosis and Venereal Disease.*
One Senior Medical Officer, 8 Medical Officers.

(4) *The Supervision of Food Supplies.*
One Senior Medical Officer, 3 Medical Officers, 1 Chemist.

(5) *General Practitioner Services.*
One Senior Medical Officer, 4 Medical Officers, 4 Divisional Medical Officers, 28 Regional Medical Officers.

(6) *Sanitary Administration in relation to Infectious Disease.*
One Senior Medical Officer, 12 Medical Officers.

(7) *Welsh Board of Health.*
One Senior Medical Officer, 3 Medical Officers, 1 Divisional and 3 Regional Medical Officers.

To add Factory Hygiene and School Hygiene to these would give uniformity of conception, and should obviate the possibility of divergent practice in the various sub-departments. But divergent practice is not the only, or the chief risk. There are others even within a single Department. The compartments may be too water-tight, and inter-communications may involve delay and "red tape" as much as if some of the compartments were in Government offices other than the Ministry of Health. There is the further "narrow neck of bottle" risk which is the curse of many branches of

Government. The chief head of a Department, be he secretarial or technical, if conscientious desires to have touch with the numerous important points of policy which arise weekly if not daily. If he fails to retain a fair amount of touch with detail, he ceases to possess that practical knowledge without which it is difficult to assess the relative value of the innovations needed to keep a system "live." If he overloads himself with detail, initiative in policy is endangered. These points are indicated not as settling the case for and against central unification of all health services; but as showing that the point cannot be settled on a merely academic basis. One is tempted to repeat the hackneyed words of Pope:

> "For forms of Government let fools contest,
> Whate'er is best administered is best."

But, notwithstanding this ejaculation, on balance one cannot doubt that there should eventually be a greater degree of central unification, while meanwhile friendly conferences are preventing friction, securing co-operation, and helping to obviate hiatuses in the health work common to several Departments. This is an easy achievement when intensely parochial (intra-departmental) proclivities are kept in restraint.

Any hesitation that may be entertained as to immediate action for unification of Central Government health functions, disappears when we consider the matter from the standpoint of local executive action *by the large public health authorities.* The great need of the Ministry of Health, of the

Factory Department of the Home Office, and of the Board of Education (in its medical and almost certainly in its non-medical work) is a large amount of devolution. The central departments are shackled and confined and rendered relatively less useful by their detailed checking of minute details in the education and poor law services, and in the public health and medical services where grants are given. The exact measures needed to secure devolution on a large scale need not be discussed here, except that they imply a large measure of trust in the county councils and county borough councils. Even if it be assumed that efficiency would temporarily suffer, inefficient responsible local government is preferable to the mere mechanical fulfilment of central regulations (see also page 113).

Chapter IX

OTHER CENTRAL HEALTH AUTHORITIES:

B. The Board of Education

Without the public elementary education which has been universally provided in Great Britain since 1870, the success already achieved in public health would have been impossible; for it depends more perhaps than on any other factor on the general enlightenment of the public, and especially on the enlightenment and consequent activities of the representatives of the public in Parliament, in the Central Government, and on Sanitary Authorities, Boards of Guardians, and Local Education Authorities.

An early evidence of this enlightenment and of the increasing sensitiveness of the public conscience was seen in the safeguarding of children. As early as 1747 scandals arising out of the poor law apprentice system called for legislation; in 1788 children of tender age were prohibited from sweeping chimneys. In 1842 a master sweep was prohibited from taking apprentices under 16 years of age.

Factory Acts beginning from 1802 were passed to prevent overwork of children, and from 1833 children under 13 years of age who were workers had to spend two hours daily in school. This was raised to three hours in 1844. It is a long stride from the beginnings of legislation to protect children, to the Children's Charter—The Children Act, 1908—containing numerous enactments for the protection of children, piloted through Parliament by Mr. (now Sir) Herbert Samuel; and to Mr. H. A. L. Fisher's Education Act of 1918, which provided that children under 12 years of age shall not be employed, and that children between 12 and 14 (the age at which compulsory full-time school attendance now ceases) shall not be employed on Sundays for more than two hours, on school days before the close of school hours, and on any day before 6 a.m. or after 8 p.m.

Voluntary effort provided some education for children in the early part of the 19th Century; and in 1833 the Treasury authorised an annual grant of £20,000 for school building. This was raised to £30,000 in 1839, when the Committee of Council on Education was appointed.

The greatest step forward was W. E. Forster's Education Act, 1870, which first appointed school boards, directly elected by the ratepayers. In 1876 it was further enacted that "it shall be the duty of the parent of every child to cause such child to receive efficient elementary instruction in reading, writing, and arithmetic." A child was defined as from 5-14 years of age. In 1880 attendance at school became compulsory; in 1887, as a natural corollary it became free, grants being given by the Treasury to replace fees of school children. In 1893 the special education of the blind and deaf was made compulsory.

In 1902 the powers of School Boards were transferred to Local Education Authorities, who number

317. These Education Authorities at this time ceased to be directly elected; but the County Council, County Borough Council, or other Urban Sanitary Authority large enough to be constituted an independent Education Authority became the Local Education Authority, its Education Committee consisting in part of members of the Local Authority and in part of members co-opted from without.

Medical inspection of schools and scholars was preceded by a number of events gradually leading up to it. For many years previously the duty had been imposed on local medical officers of health of inspecting the sanitary circumstances of school life, and their duties as regards infectious diseases necessarily kept them in close touch with problems of school attendance and child health.

The Acts of Parliament as to Blind and Deaf Children, 1893, and as to the Education of Defective and Epileptic Children, 1899, had increased both central and local knowledge of certain aspects of school hygiene. The Boer War ending in 1900 drew marked attention—as did still more the Great War of 1914-18—to the physical defects of many of our soldiers. Several Committees and Commissions were appointed, of which the most enlightening were the Royal Commission on Physical Training in Scotland, 1903, and the Inter-Departmental Committee on Physical Deterioration, 1904, the former of which especially, and both of them, did much to hasten the general installation of medical inspection of school children. In a number of towns pioneer work had been done in the medical inspection of school children prior to its central

K

organisation, notably in Bradford; and in a few towns school clinics had been started. In addition the advocacy of the feeding of underfed school children resulted in 1906 in the passing of the Education (Provision of Meals) Act, which empowered Local Education Authorities to take such steps as they think fit for feeding the children in attendance at public elementary schools in their area.

These events were followed by the enactment of the Education (Administrative Provisions) Act, 1907, which imposed the following duty and conferred the following power on Local Education Authorities :—

> " The duty to provide for the medical inspection of children immediately before, or at the time of, or as soon as possible after, their admission to a public elementary school, and on such other occasions as the Board of Education direct, and the power to make such arrangements as may be sanctioned by the Board of Education for attending to the health and physical condition of the children educated in Public Elementary Schools."

As medical inspection and the action following on it form an important branch of public health work, the power thus conferred and the duty imposed should have been initiated and supervised by the Local Government Board, as the Central Health Authority. There was and is strong reason for making the Local Public Health Committee and the Local Education Committee jointly responsible for the local execution of the work, in order that, as pointed out on page 136, educationists and hygienists might both actively engage in it. That advantage would have similarly resulted from conference between the Central Public Health Authority and the Board of Education on points of policy is evident, though the work of supervision was necessarily in the main a problem of public health. Under the separatist arrangements that were made, there followed a rapid development of a new and independently administered public health service, especially in the central government.

The "Memorandum on Medical Inspection of Children in Public Elementary Schools" (Circ. 576) issued by the Board of Education 22nd November, 1907, was admirably definite in its statement that the administration of the Education (Administrative Provisions) Act "should rest upon a broad basis of public health," that it should also use "to the utmost extent the existing machinery of medical and sanitary administration, developing and supplementing it as required, rather than supplanting it by bringing into existence new agencies, partially redundant and possibly competing." It was added that the Board (of Education) "view the whole subject of school hygiene not as a speciality or as a group of specialities existing by and of themselves but as an integral factor in the health of the nation. The application of this principle requires that the work of medical inspection should be carried out in intimate conjunction with the Public Health Authorities and under the direct supervision of the medical officer of health." The memorandum went on to say: "the advantages of such unification of the Public Health services have already been recognised by the Inter-Departmental Committee on Medical Inspection and the Feeding of School Children, and also by the Local Government Board, who specifically require every medical officer of health to report officially upon matters relating to the sanitary condition of all schools including 'action taken by the Sanitary Authority in relation to the health of the scholars and for preventing the spread of infectious disease.' "

This memorandum stated so concisely the unity of school medical work and of public health administrative work that we may advantageously give further extracts from it. Thus "efficiency and economy require an organic relationship between the daily work of the school authority and of the authority responsible for the administration of the wider branches of public health. . . . Conversely this organic relationship will provide increased opportunity and facilities for the medical officer of health to study all the conditions affecting the health of the community at all age periods, and will bring him into closer touch with the personal hygiene of the population." And the last sentence of the memorandum ran as follows: "In all steps taken the progressive unification of the medical services and the needs and circumstances of each community must continually be borne in mind."

The present position as between the Board of Education and the Ministry of Health has already been mentioned (page 103).

Influence of School Medical Inspection on the Public Health.—The good done by systematic medical inspection of school children represents one of the greatest advances in public health. Without attempting any detailed description the following points may be noted :—

(1) There has been gradually established a school medical staff of over 800 doctors engaged in routine school medical work, and nearly 500 engaged in special work (ophthalmic, aural, etc.). In addition there are already a large number of dentists engaged in dental treatment.

(2) For the treatment of school children in 1923 308 out of the 317 education authorities had more or less provision for medical treatment of one or more ailments, including special clinics, references to hospitals, provision of spectacles, etc.

(3) More than half the children found on medical inspection to be defective are now receiving treatment. It does not follow that this treatment is adequate or covers all the needs; or that school nurses and Care Committees are adequate to the requirements for visiting the homes and following up cases; and the extent of the disabilities to be combated may be gathered from the following figures (Annual Report of Chief Medical Officer of Board of Education, 1917) :—

In the years 1913-15 the number of boys and girls leaving school found to be defective were :—

	Per cent.
Uncleanliness of body	5
Ear disease	2
Defective hearing	3-5
Heart disease	4-6
Malnutrition	11
Defective vision	12-20
Diseases of nose and throat	18-20
Dental caries	67-72

These percentages, which can only be approximate, deal with children most of whom have been at school for eight or nine years, and although the percentage of defects decreases, one can realise the greatly extended medical work—and the vast preventive work—still needed. Much of the work needed to reduce these percentages is required for defects or disease arising before school life began. But already there is marked and general improvement in the cleanliness and healthiness of school children. The increased cleanliness of school children has had the additional value of raising the standard of domestic cleanliness. The pressure brought to bear by school doctors, nurses and teachers and by After-care Committees has secured the treatment of many thousands of school children, who without such treatment would be rendered relatively inadequate to the needs of adult life. Furthermore, far from diminishing the range of parental responsibility, such action has extended its scope, and has introduced parents into the partnership between them and official organisations which must exist and extend if the best obtainable in public health is to be obtained.

That the partnership and indeed the identity between the general range of public health work and workers and that of the school medical service will become more complete in the future is quite certain; and this can be secured without any sacrifice of the vital interest which Education Committees and school teachers have in the physical training, in the personal hygiene, and in the general welfare of the children in their charge.

Chapter X

THE MINISTRY OF HEALTH IN RELATION TO LOCAL AUTHORITIES

The Ministry of Health has in its charge a larger range of public health activities than its predecessor, the Local Government Board, though, as already shown, it does not deal with all central public health problems, and it is not concerned solely with these problems, but also with other problems affecting local government.

Its efficiency as will be seen in subsequent chapters is seriously hampered by the inchoate condition of the local medical work under Insurance Committees and Poor Law Guardians. There can be little improvement until the various branches of official local medical and hygienic work are unified and come under a single local authority.

This fact is well known. It has been repeatedly urged by those possessing the necessary administrative knowledge, and the following quotation from a pamphlet issued by the Ministry of Reconstruction, 1919 ("*Public Health*, II. *The Present Problem and the Ministry of Health*") echoes this skilled knowledge:—

> "Escape from the present impasse depends upon the general reform of the system of local administration. . . .
>
> "The creation of an authority (with the

> express function of undertaking the care of the people's health as a whole) is the object of the Ministry of Health Bill—no light undertaking—still a means to an end rather than an end in itself. . . .
>
> " The difficult question of the future structure of our local health organisation . . . is the first and most bounden duty of the Minister (of Health) to take in hand upon his creation."

Looking at the problem from the standpoint of the different local authorities it is stated in the same document:

> " No proposal can be made at the present time for the extension or acquisition of powers by any one set of authorities without an outcry from some other set of authorities that their province is being touched upon."

The only way out is a root and branch reform of local government. It may be hoped that the Royal Commission on Local Government now sitting will succeed in inducing the Government and Parliament at last to take their courage in their hands and to commence this herculean task. Without this a Ministry of Health must continue relatively ineffective.

One important anomaly in existing arrangements has arisen as the natural result of the gradual evolution of local authorities. Poor Law Guardians were functioning before Sanitary Authorities came into being, and the control of the official machinery for providing public vaccination was placed and has remained with them. A similar course was followed when, on the passing of the Registration of Births and Deaths Act in 1836, local registrars of births, deaths, and marriages were appointed.

As a rule the local public vaccinators were also district medical officers under the Poor Law, while the local registrar of births who was also appointed by the Board of Guardians supplied the vaccination officer of the same authority with the names of infants born, thus starting the process for securing infantile vaccination. The public vaccinator who provides free infantile vaccination is still under the local jurisdiction of the Board of Guardians; but the Ministry of Health and its predecessors the Privy Council and Local Government Board have for many years inspected the work of these vaccinators by means of their medical inspectors, and thus ensured a fairly high standard of vaccination. Grants given by the Treasury to public vaccinators are made conditional on the achievement of this standard.

Although the local registrars of marriages, births and deaths are appointed by the Boards of Guardians, their work after appointment is regulated solely by the General Register Office, Somerset House, the central bureau of the English vital statistics, which in its turn, though it is to some extent autonomous, is now a department of the Ministry of Health.

These registrars are a good illustration—apart from their initial appointment—of an admirably working local machinery controlled solely by the Central Government. It is work which requires meticulous care in the details of registration, and strict uniformity in every parish in the country. Copies of each entry in the register have to be sent to Somerset House, the officials of the central office conducting the rare prosecutions required in the event of false certification, etc. There is evidently in this case little if any call for intervention by the local representatives of the public, though any representations from these to the General Register Office would receive immediate attention.

The local supervision of vaccination and the appointment of local registrars of births and deaths should, it is generally agreed, be transferred to County Councils and County Borough Councils, thus securing large-scaled and fairly equalised local administration, in which the operation of local prejudice against measures for securing vaccination, and local inefficiency will be minimised.

The scheme shown on page 51 shows that there are 1,727 sanitary authorities, 635 poor law authorities, and 317 local education authorities. It may be added that a given area of poor law administration often embraces a considerable number of sanitary areas, and that in a county borough not infrequently the unit of poor law differs most embarrassingly from that of public health administration.

The confusion for educational health administration is even more marked. In some counties the education authority for the entire county is the County Council; in others there are enclaves of separate education authorities. These and allied anomalies are inimical to economical and efficient public health administration. Thus in county work notifications of births may be received by the medical officer of health of the small local authority or of the County Council; and visits of health visitors may be organised on a county or on a local scale. Notifications of puerperal fever from doctors are received by the local and not the county medical officer of health (except by courtesy), but the latter receives such notifications in the cases attended by midwives, and has to arrange for the necessary investigation and precautionary measures.

Tuberculosis work is organised on a county scale, but the local medical officer of health has duties in regard to each notified case, which overlap with those of the tuberculosis officer of the County Council.

Further illustrations of local inco-ordination.

(1) The fact that several local authorities deal with mental defectives, e.g. paupers and school children, shows the continued confusion between duties of the Board of Guardians, the local Education Committee, and the Sanitary Authority.

(2) An insured person who is pregnant can claim attendance from her panel doctor, but not for the confinement, i.e. attendance at labour or within ten days afterwards in respect of any condition arising therefrom. At her confinement she receives a monetary benefit from the Society with which she is insured, but provides her own doctor. She may also receive assistance in connection with the Maternity and Child Welfare scheme of a local authority.

(3) The panel doctor treats an insured patient for ordinary ailments not beyond the average skill of a medical practitioner. This may include partial

treatment, for instance, of venereal disease; but for these diseases, as also for acute infectious diseases, separate provision may be made by the Guardians, and is made by the County Council or County Borough Council.

(4) A school child may be treated for adenoids or ringworm at a school clinic under the Education Committee of a non-county Authority, for tuberculosis under a scheme of a County Council, for scarlet fever by the local Sanitary Authority, and if destitute may be treated for any disease by the Board of Guardians.

(5) A school child with tuberculous hip may be received into an institution controlled by the Local Education Authority; if younger or if beyond school age he may be treated by the Board of Guardians or the Public Health Authority.

Illustrations might be multiplied showing that in present circumstances some form of health service is provided by the following local authorities, not all of which have co-terminous areas, and which act in large measure in segregation from each other.

For the insured population, by the Insurance Committee of the County or County Borough;

For children of school age, by the Education Authority;

For the destitute of all ages, by the Board of Guardians;

For discharged and disabled war pensioners, by the Local War Pensions Committee;

For the insane and mentally defective poor, by the Local Education Authority, by the Defective Children's Committee of the County Council or

County Borough Council, or by the Board of Guardians.

The defects of local administration will receive further consideration in the chapters dealing with Poor Law and Insurance Administration; but it is convenient to state here the general lines of reform that are required.

There is a consensus of opinion on the part of the vast majority of those experienced in the work of local administration, and unanimously on the part of various Royal Commissions and Governmental Committees, that there is needed reform in three chief directions:—

1st. The local governing functions now divided among a number of local authorities—whose duties in many particulars overlap or even conflict—should be concentrated in one local authority for each area, which will form its Local Parliament or Council, Committees having relegated to them executive action for certain definite functions as for instance

Health and Medical Treatment,
Relief of Destitution,
Education,
Finance, and other Committees.

The Health Committee's functions in populous areas may advantageously be sub-divided under various Sub-Committees as those of

Sanitation,
Maternity and Child Welfare Work,
Tuberculosis and Venereal Disease Work,
Hospital and Sanatorium Administration,
School Medical Work.

On the last named Committee the Education Committee should receive liberal representation.

2nd. Outside county borough administration larger units of administration are required. County boroughs in nearly every instance have a population exceeding 50,000. Outside these county boroughs there is needed a closer relationship between each County Council and the sanitary authorities within its area, and the number of these authorities should be severely reduced.

It is especially in connection with the major health services that the larger units of administration are required. In such matters as the following, which are specially enumerated in a recent Report to the Scottish Board of Health by Consultative Councils on "A Reformed Local Authority for Health and Public Assistance," the need for larger units of administration is clamant, smaller units implying generally inferior administration, and expenditure which is excessive for results obtained.

Housing and Town Planning;
Hospital and other institutional services;
Infectious diseases (including tuberculosis and venereal diseases);
Vaccination;
Medical Benefit under the Insurance Acts;
Maternity and Child Welfare;
Medical Inspection and treatment of School Children;
Food and meat inspection and milk supply;
Contagious Diseases of Animals Acts;
Water supply;
Drainage;

Prevention of rivers pollution.

There is need to overhaul the country county by county, arranging for a gradual combination of districts, and for the abolition of the smaller units. It would be a good practical rule to abolish all sanitary districts too small to employ advantageously a whole time medical officer of health. This would reduce their number by at least one-half. There is needed also a closer relationship between county and district health administration, to secure co-ordination and co-operation in both the major and the minor branches of administration.

3rd. The duties of Boards of Guardians should be transferred to County Councils and County Borough Councils as recommended unanimously by the Royal Commission on the Poor Laws, and by the Maclean Committee (Report of the Local Government Sub-Committee of the Ministry of Reconstruction, 1917 (Cd. 8917)). This Committee comprised many of the members of the previous Poor Law Royal Commission, and can fairly be regarded as having arranged a practical compromise on which members who wrote the Majority and Minority Reports of that Commission unanimously agreed.

The report of this Committee was issued in the year 1917; and it has been recently urged by representatives of Poor Law Authorities that it is now out-of-date and that the entire question of the relation of poor law to public health local activities requires to be re-considered. On the medical side there appears to be no ground for this contention. Poor Law Guardians in many unions have improved their arrangements for the treatment of the sick and even made arrangements for the treatment in their institutions of persons not technically destitute. But there remain serious and permanent difficulties in the treatment of the sick poor, so long as this remains in the hands of authorities concerned in the sparing monetary relief of the destitute; and this association is an effective bar to the treatment of the sick on public health principles.

The new fact is the inordinate amount of unemployment since the Great War, which renders it impracticable for many Boards of Guardians to meet the financial liability involved. This it may at once be said is a valid reason for making Insurance against Unemployment effective over a long series of years, when it will probably become monetarily solvent; but it does not furnish a satisfactory reason for delaying the transfer of the duties of Boards of Guardians to larger authorities, which would be able to classify the destitute needing institutional treatment satisfactorily, and to transfer the medical and hygienic care of the poor to public health authorities concerned in prevention as well as in treatment.

Schemes for county boroughs and for London are given in this Report. Without entering into further detail, I give here the recommendations of this Committee in their own words:—

> "We recommend the abolition of the Boards of Guardians and of the Poor Law Union, and the merging of all the functions of the Poor Law Authorities in those of the County Council and

the County Borough Council, subject to the necessary modifications set out in our Schemes below for London and the other administrative counties.

"We recommend that—

(*a*) The provision at the expense of the rates, with or without Exchequer Grants, for the sick and infirm (including maternity and infancy and the aged requiring institutional care, and all institutions appropriated to any of these) should be made by the Council under Public Health Acts suitably extended. The Council should organise such preventive and curative treatment as the cases individually require by means of their specialised institutions and medical staff.

(*b*) The provision for all children able to attend school (including residential and special schools of all kinds) should be regarded as predominantly a matter of educational training, and should be made by the Local Education Authority under the Education Acts suitably extended.

(*c*) The provision for the mentally deficient, and for persons of unsound mind whether certified or not, including all institutions appropriated to these classes, should be made by the Council under the Lunacy and Mental Deficiency Acts, suitably extended, and through the Committee or Committees administering their powers under these Acts.

"We recommend that the County or County Borough Council, as the case may be, should be required to appoint, in substitution for the existing authorities under the Poor Law and under the Unemployed Workmen Act, a new Committee, to be entitled 'The Prevention of Unemployment and Training Committee,' formed on the lines of the Education Committee, and including representatives of Employers Associations and of Organised Labour. The Committee should exercise the powers of the Council as to (i) preventing unemployment (so far as practicable, and subject to service requirements and due economy) by procuring such a rearrangement of the Council's works and services as to regularise the local demand for labour; (ii) facilitating through the Employment Exchanges the finding of situations; (iii) making use of any form of educational training in co-operation as much as possible with the Education Committee; (iv) assisting migration; and (v) creating and administering, whether by themselves or in federation with other Local Authorities, any specialised provision of the kind required by the unemployed.

"We recommend that the County or County Borough Council, as the case may be, should be required to appoint a new Committee, to be styled 'the Home Assistance Committee,' formed on the lines of the Education Committee (including persons experienced in the work to be done, and, in the first instance, some who have been members of Poor Law Authorities), which should be charged with (i) the duty of making the necessary enquiries into the economic circumstances of applicants for or recipients of any form of assistance in money, kind, or service, wholly or partly provided out of rates or taxes, eligibility for which is dependent on the pecuniary need of the person or family concerned, or for which payment is legally recoverable; (ii) general supervision of recipients of such assistance and their dependants; (iii) the administration of all such assistance in money or kind given in the home of the applicant; (iv) the exercise of the powers of the guardians of acquiring the rights and powers of parents as regards any children maintained by them who are orphans or whose parents are unfit to have the care of them; (v) the duty of seeking in co-operation with the appropriate committee institutional treatment for any applicant or the dependant of any applicant for whom such treatment is required; (vi) the recovery from persons liable by law of expenses in respect of accommodation, maintenance, treatment, and services rendered; and (vii) the duty of keeping a register (which should not be open to public inspection) of all families within the area, any member of which is in receipt of assistance as above defined, together with particulars of such assistance.

"We recommend that the officers of the Poor Law Authorities should be transferred to the County and County Borough Councils under schemes to be approved by the Local Government Board, the Councils and the officers both having an option as to transfer; and that suitable provision should be made for the adequate compensation of all such officers as may suffer direct pecuniary loss owing either to abolition of office or to a diminution or loss of emoluments in fees, salary, or allowances. The tenure of office and all rights of superannuation of existing officers who are transferred should be fully protected.

"We recommend that the property and liabilities of all Poor Law Authorities should be allocated among the Councils concerned, or any combinations of them, by the Local Government Board, or by some person appointed by them, after these Councils have had an opportunity of effecting a mutual arangement.

"We recommend that pending the amendment of the law relating to the valuation of property, the power of appointing the Assessment Committees should be transferred to the County and County Borough Councils, and throughout London to the Metropolitan Borough Councils. The Councils should determine through which of their committees, not being the Home Assistance Committee, they will administer any functions of the Boards of Guardians or combinations of Boards of Guardians (including those under the Vaccination and Births and Deaths Registration Acts) not already specified; provided that all *functions relating to Health*, Education, the provision for Lunacy and Mental Deficiency and the provision for Unemployment respectively should *be administered exclusively under the several Acts relating thereto*, suitably extended, and through the Committees dealing with such Acts."

Following on this report, the then Government gave a pledge in the House of Commons " of adherence to the recommendations of this Committee and of an intention to proceed in the matter as soon as possible."

In 1919, when the Ministry of Health Bill was introduced, the Government apparently was not in a position to proceed with local public health reform, the more urgent as well as the more difficult portion of the problem; but they adopted the probably unique procedure of stating that it was " the intention of this Act " in the event of future legislation to make the transfers of duties of Boards of Guardians indicated above. This still remains to be done.

For certain purposes, e.g. joint sewerage schemes, joint supply of water for large areas, and institutional provision, it may sometimes be necessary to institute special groupings of authorities, larger than county councils and county borough councils; but for the majority of public health operations there is no reason why the grouping into counties and county boroughs should not be adopted as the basis of reformed local public health administration (see also page 93).

Chapter XI

PUBLIC HEALTH ADMINISTRATION IN RELATION TO SANITARY CIRCUMSTANCES

PRECEDING chapters have illustrated many of the practical problems with which ministration of health, central and local, is concerned.

The list of contents of the chief clauses of the Public Health Act, 1875, page 25 , shows the importance attached in the earlier stages of public health progress to environmental as distinguished from personal hygiene. The distinction here made can only be partial, for a large part of the environment of each person consists in the personal influence of parents, nurses, teachers and companions. But in the earlier history of public health, sanitary questions as to food supply, water supply, scavenging, drainage and sewerage affecting the masses of the people, and capable of being put right in large measure without the exercise of individual hygiene, were the chief subjects of legislative enactment and administrative action.

The duties of the medical officer of health as prescribed for many years by the central Ministry of Health (page 40) lay chief stress on the prevention of epidemic diseases, and after this on supervision of food supplies, and on the sanitary circumstances including housing conditions of the district; and in his annual report the medical officer of health is expected to report under the headings set out on page 46.

The above-mentioned environmental evils provoke disease and depress the standard of health; and they still maintain their place as the elementary and more urgent requirements of sanitary administration. For this reason, and because subsequent chapters will be concerned more particularly with the social and medical problems of health ministration, it is appropriate to introduce here a short sketch of some of the activities involved in the sanitary control of a community.

The elementary requirements may be stated to be

(1) Wholesome food;

(2) A pure and adequate water supply;

(3) Prompt and complete removal of excretory products (urine and fæces) from the vicinity of dwellings;

(4) The prevention of aerial pollution by

(*a*) Undue aggregation of persons in crowded conditions;

(*b*) Industrial or other dust;

(*c*) Smoke, cutting off natural sunlight.

For a more complete enumeration of sanitary circumstances see page 45.

Over each of the above evils Public Health Acts give control in greater or less degree; and through such control exercised by sanitary authorities, immense improvement in public health has been achieved.

Protection of food.—This is an elementary requirement of public health administration, and by the Public Health Acts power is given to the medical officer of health and the sanitary inspector to enter and examine any animal or other food which is being prepared or is exposed for sale for human food. Powers of seizure of unsound or diseased food are given, and a magistrate is empowered to order its destruction. Prosecution of the vendor may follow. There are various by-laws for the regulation of slaughter-houses, but the use of public abattoirs is not enforced, and in their absence completely satisfactory supervision of animal foods is not secured.

Milk is the food which most of all needs protection and there are enactments and regulations both as regards dirty milk and milk from diseased animals, and also as to adulteration of milk by the addition of chemicals, the addition of water or the abstraction of cream. Preservatives are forbidden in milk. The sanitary officers have the power of inspecting dairies and persons employed in them; and all dairies must be registered.

For further details on the above subjects and as to adulteration of foods other than milk, appropriate text-books in hygiene can be consulted.

Water is one of the prime necessaries of life, and impure water has caused devastating epidemics of cholera, dysentery, and typhoid fever. In this country such epidemics are now rare, owing to the care taken to protect municipal and other supplies of water from contamination at their source and during the transit to the domestic circle. The sums spent on communal water supplies are gigantic. In England and Wales in the year 1913-14 loans amounting to £2,161,555 and of £3,259,166 in the preceding year were sanctioned for expenditure on waterworks by local authorities. The legal provisions for protecting water supplies will be found in various legal handbooks.

Scavenging was one of the earliest of provisions in sanitary law. It has become almost perfected in large towns. The water carriage of sewage has greatly diminished the danger to health implied in the retention of domestic refuse about the dwelling; but accumulations of non-excremental refuse remain a detriment to domestic comfort, and large public expenditure is regularly incurred in its removal.

House Drainage and Municipal Sewerage are the subject of numerous enactments, which in most towns have reduced the risks of excremental poisoning, with one exception, to a low ebb. Water closets are the rule in most areas, and elaborate systems of disposal of sewage are provided. The one great exception is the risk of fæcal contamination of an infant's food from dirty napkins or from the unwashed hands of the mother or nurse who prepares this food. Flies are dangerous as contaminators of food chiefly when they have previously been in contact with fæcal matter, which in this country, with the exceptions named above, seldom occurs in most districts.

Dusty Occupations are a serious peril to health. In factories their control comes within the domain of the Home Office, and the local health officers can exercise little or no control over them. There is need in this respect for utilisation by the Home Office of the local sanitary inspector.

Smoke Prevention is still in its infancy, though some improvement has been secured. The limitation of powers of sanitary authorities to the emission of "black smoke" and the further limitation of this power to factories has made progress difficult.

Overcrowding is an evil against which energetic action has been taken throughout the whole course of sanitary administration. It is an evil most difficult to control; for the ordinary action under the nuisance clauses of the Public Health Acts may merely mean removal from a known to an unknown crowded dwelling. Some good is done; but when housing provision is scant, this is but little. Too little regard has been paid to the distinction between crowding of healthy persons and crowded association of the sick—especially the tuberculous sick—with the healthy. Action for separation of sick from healthy is supremely urgent, and notification returns often enable this to be done. It has been too little secured in the management of cases of open tuberculosis.

The control of overcrowding is part of the larger question of *Housing*, the most serious social problem of to-day. The legislation on housing is legion. It is part of the social incubus resulting from the rapid change of England from a chiefly agricultural to a chiefly manufacturing country, from rural to urban life, without adequate building by-laws or sanitation. There is a problem of "over-housing," in the sense of overcrowding of houses on area, as well as of "overcrowding," and much of our modern difficulty in housing has been caused by this excessive closeness of packing of houses on area, with consequent interference with perflation of air, access of light and sunlight, and facilities for sanitary conveniences. In the last fifteen years greatly increased efforts have been made to limit this overcrowding of houses on area, not only by means of building by-laws, but also by town planning schemes, which still need further encouragement. Too little has been done in large schemes for the clearance of insanitary areas. The proportion of overcrowded dwellings is immensely greater in urban than in rural houses; and the evils of overcrowding, even given equal proportions of overcrowding in rural and in urban areas, are much more serious in towns, owing to the more frequent and more extensive personal inter-communications and consequent transmission of various infections.

The course of legislation, Act following Act at intervals of a few years, cannot be traced here. It may be stated generally that sanitary authorities have been empowered on the certificate of their medical officer of health to close dwelling-houses, and if the conditions are beyond repair to order their demolition; also to condemn insanitary areas of houses, giving compensation to the owners of the property concerned.

Houses wear out like human beings; but unlike the latter they remain after their utility and life have passed. Such houses can be dealt with singly; but where houses were originally too densely aggregated, interfering with access of light and air, wider destruction is called for.

In order that this policy may be pursued without hardship, new houses are required, and Sanitary

Authorities have been empowered under certain conditions to erect dwelling-houses for the working-class. The Housing, Town Planning, etc. Act of 1909 included important new clauses, which were extended in the Housing Act of 1919. This Act commences with a declaration that it shall be the duty of every local authority to consider the needs of its area with respect to the provision of houses for the working classes, and requires these authorities to submit schemes for providing such houses to the Local Government Board (now the Ministry of Health). The more recent housing legislation, subsidising the erection of working classes' houses cannot be summarised here. The Act of 1924 proposes the erection of two or three million houses suitable for the occupation of the working classes, during a period of fifteen years; these houses are to be let to their occupants at uneconomic rents; and the loss will fall therefore partly on the ratepayer, but chiefly on the taxpayer. Whether such a departure from economic considerations is justified is a debatable point. The terrible amount of National Debt incurred by the first efforts after the Great War in this direction throws a lurid light on such action. If at all, non-economic action must be justified by the existence of exceptional circumstances not likely to recur, and it is doubtful if this can be done.

We may properly ask whether there is no alternative policy? If the excessive cost of building dwelling houses cannot be reduced—it might be reduced given an adequate output of work and an absence of commercial rings for profiteering—

then the alternative is to ascertain whether money now spent or wasted in other directions cannot be diverted towards paying for expensive but indispensable housing. If this country were like the United States "to go dry" the money would be at once forthcoming; and short of this, by reduction of our National Drink Bill by one-half, the housing difficulty would be solved. As Dr. James Niven remarks in his "Observations on the History of Public Health Effort in Manchester," 1923:

> "Can there be any doubt that the liquor trade paralyses the hands of the social reformer and keeps the people poor?"

Chapter XII

DESTITUTION AND THE PUBLIC HEALTH

In this and following chapters the word " poverty " is used in the sense of indigence or destitution, for which some form of material aid is required if injury to health or to some other essential element in well-being is to be avoided.

The need for relief of poverty has always been realised, in earlier days to avoid social anarchy, and more recently because the intimate relation between poverty, disease and social inefficiency has become appreciated. Such relief has therefore always been one of the most important duties of civil administration. History is full of attempts to deal with this problem, ranging from the old Roman *panem et circenses* to the drastic legislation of the VI Edwardian and Elizabethan reigns.

It is generally agreed that indigence is undesirable, and in the public interest ought, if practicable, to be removed. Is this practicable, and if so to what extent? The attempt to answer this question involves a study of perhaps the most important of public health problems, a problem which penetrates deeply into the whole social fabric. It is in short a social study in causation. The answer of social workers to the question what are the underlying causes of poverty will differ according to the personality of the investigator. If he is connected with a religious organisation he may lay stress on moral dereliction and depravity as a cause of indigence; if a temperance reformer, alcoholic indulgence is likely to figure largely in his statistics; if a eugenist of the positive and dogmatic school he will be confident, in the words of Tennyson's "Northern Farmer," that "the poor in the lump be bad," that there is some inherent weakness in their character, and that destitution in reality constitutes a sorting out of the undesirable from the desirable. According to the bias of the observer, ignorance; shiftlessness and inefficiency; crime and dishonesty; drink; immorality; gambling; insufficiently paid employment; lack or insufficiency of occupation; death or sickness of the breadwinner; unhealthy occupation; accident; physical defects; old age, or a large family, will appear as the chief cause of indigence. In studying the causation of Poverty certain fundamental considerations need to be borne in mind.

1st. *Poverty* (defined as above) *is a complex, comprising many elements*, variously combined in the production of the aggregate phenomenon; and each case of poverty must be studied individually if the correct diagnosis is to be made and the appropriate remedy applied. To suppose that the direct bestowment of money on the impoverished is an efficient remedy is contrary to reason; though if a family have insufficient earnings this palliative must inevitably be employed, pending better measures. The impoverishment may be the result of intemperance, or gambling, or improvidence. Here the giving of money may intensify the evil, although in practice one may be morally compelled to depart in such a case from strictly economic conduct. Thus the children of a drunken parent are given school meals, in cases in which the reformation of the parent cannot be brought about; the greater need being to protect the child from the consequences of protracted malnutrition.

The illustration of poverty due to drunkenness may be further studied. The intemperance may have been favoured by initial weakness of moral fibre of the future drunkard. It has been fostered by evil social habits, especially that of treating; the way has been prepared for it by the lack of moral training in the home and school; it is favoured by overwork, by unsatisfactory housing, by a shiftless wife who cannot cook satisfying food; and the excessive number of public houses, the inadequate restriction of hours of sale of drink, the absence of Sunday closure of public houses, have made it difficult for a weak man to resist the temptations of an exigent habit.

The American plan of prohibition is a "short cut" out of this complex of contributory factors of intemperance, and it has been remarkably successful in the greater part of the United States. It could not have been so, had it not represented the vast preponderance of public opinion; and the social reformer in this country, while educating public opinion in favour of restrictive measures for the incontinent minority, will desire to attack indigence due to intemperance along all the channels indicated above.

2nd. The relation of social problems to one

another is seldom one of mere sequence; commonly there is mutual dependance and transferability. As Emeritus Professor Dr. Peabody of Harvard University has put it, *each problem is another in disguise.* Thus the underpaid workman and his family are likely to be underfed and unsatisfactorily housed. His health fails, he loses his employment, and casual destitution becomes permanent.

Family poverty again has led to premature employment of children; their normal growth is affected detrimentally; as adults they are relatively inefficient, and thus poverty is perpetuated. The instances of vicious circles produced by and producing poverty might easily be multiplied. The evident lesson is that poverty is a problem which needs to be attacked from many points of view. In its severest forms it is among the most maleficent of sanitary evils; and to secure efficient sanitation poverty must be vigorously attacked.

As Simon put it many years ago:

> "The public health of a country means the health of its masses, and the masses will scarcely be healthy unless to their very base they be at least moderately prosperous."

Did not St. Augustine also say:

> "Thou givest bread to the hungry, but better were it, that none hungered and thou had'st none to give him"?

3rd. Poverty being a symptom complex, it is most important that in every case we should *seek to divide the consideration of poverty into that of its component parts.* Investigation on these lines enables us to particularise in our preventive efforts, while

M

remaining confident that each set of measures will help towards reducing poverty; it further promotes confidence, which is needed for complete success, in the efforts of others who are devoting themselves to other factors of poverty than the particular one in which we may have special concern.

It is not suggested that the direct relief of poverty will not directly diminish disease. Poverty commonly means over-fatigue, overcrowding, and dirt, which may be attacked by taking steps against each of these social evils, or by direct relief. Nor can it be doubted that whatever other aids are brought to bear there is likely to remain a cruel residuum of poverty, which can only be removed by direct relief of privation.

4th. The *importance of a careful analysis* of the circumstances of poverty is particularly great *when sickness accompanies it.* In such a case the interest of the community as well as of the family in question can only be met by sparing no medical or nursing or material assistance which will conduce to early restoration to economic and social efficiency. This point is essential, and it is one on which poor law administration in the past has partially failed.

In associated poverty and sickness as in other forms of indigence, a causal analysis is essential; for a large mass of sickness is preventable, and even when this is not so, the later and more severe results of sickness are often preventable when patients secure prompt and adequate treatment, in the full sense of medical supervision, good nursing, and nutrition.

Essential difference between medical and non-medical aid.—In this connection it is well to remember the fundamental difference between medical and non-medical provision at the cost of the public. This difference is embodied in the following remarks by the late Rev. Dr. Chalmers of Glasgow, which are quoted in Mr. and Mrs. Webb's "The Prevention of Destitution." Dr. Chalmers was the great apostle of voluntary charity on a parochial basis as preferable to any form of official relief; and for some years he demonstrated the practicability of this method—in which personal reserves, aid from relatives, and then voluntary help were all utilised—in his own parish in Glasgow. But he had no intention of leaving the sick poor to even systematic help by voluntary charity; and he advocated and demanded public and complete provision for the sick and for the mentally defective, and a national system of educational provision for children. The sick bodily and mentally together constitute two-thirds of our present total pauperism. He made the following far-seeing observations:

> "The distinction between . . . a public charity for the relief of indigence and a public charity for the relief of disease must not have occurred to the civilised governments of Europe, else it would have more frequently been acted on. . . . An ostensible provision for the relief of poverty creates more poverty. An ostensible provision for the relief of disease does not cause more disease. The human will is enlisted on the side of poverty by the provision which is made for it. No such provision will ever enlist the human will on the side of disease. . . . An indefinite provision for want is ever sure to multiply its objects. . . . The open

proclamation of a free entry into asylums of disease would make a clean abridgement of human misery, and bring no new or additional disease into existence. The argument against a public charity for indigence applies so little to the public charities for disease that, practically, while the former ought to be abolished, the latter, with a proper degree of regulation and watchfulness, might be encouraged to the uttermost."

It is unnecessary to argue here the question as to the relative importance of poverty and disease in the production of social misery. Beyond doubt each may, in any practical sense of the word, cause the other, but I record my own opinion that disease much oftener causes poverty than poverty disease. Poverty probably causes less disease through actual privation than it causes through uncleanliness and crowding, through ignorance of the ways and means that are available even to the poverty-stricken, and often through alcoholism. It is, of course, immensely more difficult for the poor than for the comfortably circumstanced to avoid these evils. That poverty and disease work on each other in a vicious circle is obvious. But this circle has the quality of its defect, for the circle can be broken at any point; and the practical problem in a high proportion of the total cases of poverty is concerned with the means by which it may be possible to stop people from becoming poor by preventing them from becoming or remaining sick. This is not the only way in which the problem of poverty can and ought to be attacked; but this mode of attack has not received the attention that it deserves, and it is a method which will yield a higher and a quicker return for the energy and money required than others which at present are more in the public eye.

It is not suggested that an adequate service of medical treatment and nursing will abolish poverty; but if systematically and scientifically employed, as a man of "big business" would manage any of his problems after careful investigation, the mass of poverty would be enormously reduced by such a service.

Treatment and Prevention of Disease form an Inseparable Problem.—This is especially well seen in the case of tuberculosis. Timely treatment, a liberal dietary, and an observance of hygienic regulations on the part of a consumptive suffering from early disease not only increase his prospect of recovery, but also obviate risk for his wife and children. Similarly in the treatment of syphilis, the administration of an arseno-benzol preparation not only prepares the way for cure, but also inhibits the patient's competence to infect others, by destroying the infective material in superficial lesions. The case of the acute infectious diseases need not be argued; for our great triumphs against typhus and typhoid fever could not have been secured but for the skilled combination of hospital treatment and segregation of those affected with these diseases.

Unfortunately in the past there has been an unwritten law that public health authorities, central and local, were only or at least were almost solely concerned with the prevention of infection and with such treatment as is incidental to this. It is a point of view against which medical officers of health from time to time have struggled with increasing success; child welfare and school medical work have opened out increasingly a wider outlook; and now public health authorities concern themselves with

(1) Dietetics and other branches of personal hygiene conducing to the prevention of disease and the elevation of the standard of health, e.g. in regard to rickets and various forms of malnutrition; and

(2) The treatment of various non-infectious diseases which lower efficiency or produce invalidism, e.g. adenoids, ear diseases, defects of eyesight, dental caries in expectant or nursing mothers, and so on.

Chapter XIII

POOR LAW AND PUBLIC HEALTH ADMINISTRATION

FOR many centuries the population of England increased very slowly, hunger and pestilence being "the drill-sergeant of society." In the mediæval statutes the labourer who left his parish was treated almost as a fugitive slave, this severe policy reaching its climax in the reigns of Edward VI and Elizabeth, when the "rogue, vagabond, or sturdy beggar" was liable to be branded with an R on his shoulder, and handed over to anyone who would take him. The other side of this cruelty was that the Poor Law Act of 1601 laid down a policy, not modified until 1834, which gave, while immobilising him in his own parish, to every destitute person the right to assistance. Thus in England while the vagabond could be flogged, sent to prison, or if necessary hanged (*The English Utilitarians*, by Leslie Stephen, p. 90), the resident pauper had the right to maintenance. This contrasted markedly with the Irish poor law policy; and the immobilisation of the destitute in England and their wide vagrancy in Ireland largely explains the differing history of typhus fever in the two countries.

The system of poor-relief thus developed was under the control of local Boards of Guardians, who were elected by the ratepayers of the parish.

The effect of the system was to give the labourer an inadequate fixed wage and a parochial bounty, often graduated according to the number of children in the pauper's family. Prudence was placed at a discount, a premium was placed on illegitimacy, and the moral sense of the community was depraved.

The Poor Law Amendment Act of 1834 initiated four great changes:—

(1) The Central Government obtained control over the system of local relief. (2) Smaller parishes were joined into Unions, to distribute more evenly the burden of the poor. (3) Outdoor relief to able-bodied men was forbidden (this was never entirely effective). (4) Settlement in new places was made much easier.

The great problem at that time was the question of relief for the able-bodied, who through unemployment or underpayment were unable to maintain themselves and their families. For these the only choice given was so-called complete independence or the workhouse. The report of the Royal Commission recommended the provision of distinct institutions for four classes—the aged and really impotent, children, able-bodied females, and able-bodied males. In this way it was expected, in the words of the Report, that each class would "receive an appropriate treatment; the old might enjoy their indulgences without torment from the boisterous; the children be educated; and the able-bodied subjected to such courses of labour and discipline as will repel the indolent and vicious."

So far as the able-bodied were concerned, this drastic reform destroyed the evil association between out-door or home relief and the payment of insufficient wages by farmers; and right up to the present day there has been in most Unions a steady struggle between the destitute and poor law administration, varying in severity in each Union according to the views of the particular Board of Guardians.

The greater ease of migration and the increasing development of urban industries led to overcrowding of the rural population into towns, where another set of vicious social circles was initiated. They lived in filthy cellars and tenements, their numbers enabled manufacturers to cut wages, and the mortality from typhus and other epidemics was terribly high; and relief given, when destitution was in being, failed to break the circle of evil.

Although the rigid rules as regards able-bodied paupers restricted official charity, the influence of these rules in reducing indigence was on a relatively small scale. To an uncertain extent they increased thrift; but the new, like the old machinery, did not lead to action outside the rigid limitation of relief for the able-bodied, which would help to build up disabled families or to prevent families from falling hopelessly and permanently into destitution. As a rule destitution was absolute before relief was given; and we now know that a more elastic system based on intelligent study of each case and the adoption of preventive and curative methods might often have prevented the complete breaking up of the home. The time for causal as distinguished from symptomatic treatment had not yet come; not has it yet come to the extent which is needed.

Unfortunately the promiscuity of the general

workhouse was retained. It meant the evils associated with relief in the same institution of children and adults, and of prostitutes and unmarried mothers with their first infant; to which must be added, especially in the case of rural workhouses, nursing by ignorant paupers, and inadequate and unspecialised medical care.

In the earlier years of the operation of the Poor Law Amendment Act of 1834, the Poor Law Commissioners favoured restriction of medical relief, as encouraging "resort to the poor-rates for medical relief." After 1847 there was some increase of leniency in the giving of medical relief; and in 1854 a Select Committee, before which Charles Kingsley gave evidence, recommended that this might be given "without the recipient being placed on the list of paupers."

In 1865-6 a special inquiry instituted by the *Lancet* showed that

> "We have allowed a number of establishments to grow up in the external semblance of hospitals for paupers, but in truth the whole business is a sham, a mere simulacrum of real hospital accommodation."

The Guardians of the Poor and the Local Government Board appear never to have completely freed themselves from the generalised conception that the position of the pauper must remain during the giving of relief inferior to that of the non-pauper: a sound and necessary principle when applied to the drifting able-bodied adult; but mischievous when applied to sick persons or to women and children.

All this time the number of able-bodied paupers was steadily decreasing; and the Poor Law became predominantly a national organisation for the relief of sick (including the mentally sick) poor,

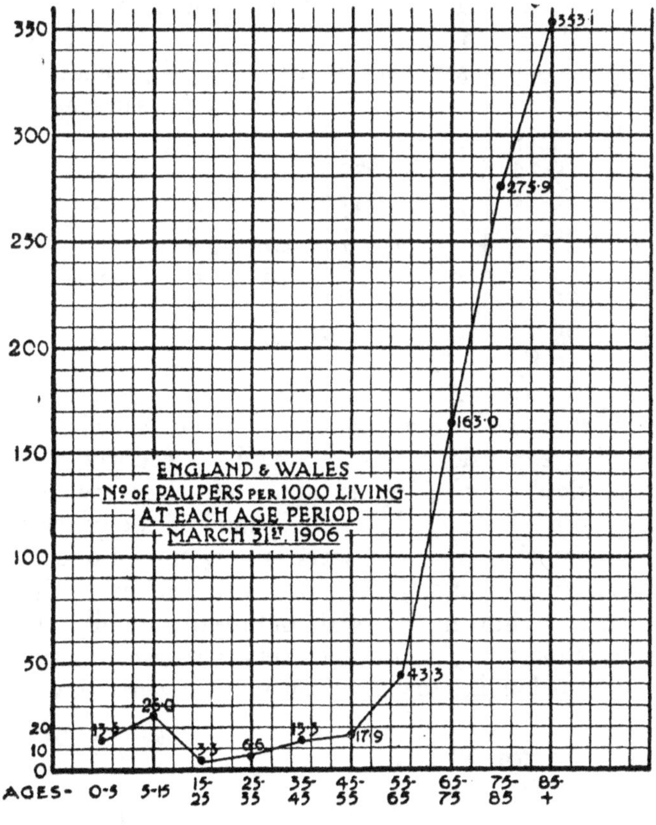

Diagram showing for England and Wales the number of Paupers of different ages on a given day in 1906 per 1,000 of the total population at these ages.

and of the aged and infirm and children. The change is indirectly indicated in the preceding diagram showing the ratio of paupers to total population at each age period in 1906, on a day on which a special census was taken. Unfortunately more recent data of the same kind cannot be given.

It will be seen that

at ages 0-5 years, 1 in 73 of the total population at the same ages.

„	5-15	„	„	38	„	„	„
„	15-25	„	„	303	„	„	„
„	25-35	„	„	151	„	„	„
„	35-45	„	„	75	„	„	„
„	45-55	„	„	56	„	„	„
„	55-65	„	„	23	„	„	„
„	65-75	„	„	6	„	„	„
„	75-85	„	„	4	„	„	„
„	85-95	„	„	3	„	„	„

in the year 1906 were in receipt of parochial relief.

Old age pensions should now have reduced the proportions at the higher ages, but they are not likely to have changed the significance of the general statement that poor law work is now chiefly one of organisation for the care of the sick (including the insane), the infirm, the aged, and destitute children.

In January, 1908, out of every 100 paupers the number belonging to each of the following groups was

	Percentage of total Paupers.
Insane and idiot poor	12.1
Sane poor :—	
(1) Aged and infirm adults	47·9
(2) Adults ordinarily able-bodied	12.9
(3) Children	25·3
(4) Casual or vagrant poor	1.8

This means that on the date mentioned at least 48 per cent. of the total paupers in England and Wales were returned as adults, mentally or physically incapacitated. The children are in the list either because they are ill, or because of the illness or death of one or both parents; temporary illness is included in many of the group (2) and of group (4).

Less than one-tenth of paupers resident in institutions are adults in health, and probably at least one-half of the so-called able-bodied men receive relief on account of their own sickness. In a contribution to the Journal of the Royal Statistical Society (Vol. lxxi, Pt. I) Dr. Basil Cook showed that in the three parishes of Bermondsey, Camberwell, and Kensington, during the months of May and June, 1907, 70 per cent. of the total indoor pauperism was due to bodily sickness. Dr. Nathan Raw after examining 4,000 cases of phthisis in a poor law infirmary in Liverpool came to the conclusion that 60 per cent. of them had become paupers owing to their illness.

The Report of the Royal Commission on the Poor Laws gave among their reasons for reform, the facts that pauperism is almost as prevalent as it was forty years ago, that expenditure on poor relief has grown out of all proportion to the number relieved, and that the Union bears no definite relation to other authorities who now perform functions which overlap the work of the Guardians. On the two first of these points some misapprehension is liable to occur. The poor law has become the chief organisation in the country for dealing with the bodily and mentally sick. The facts that the number of indoor paupers per 1,000 of population has increased, and the number of total paupers has not greatly declined, is no indication of a serious national condition. On the contrary the only sound inference is that the public are realising more and more the value of poor law infirmaries as hospitals for the general population, and are claiming their right as ratepayers to their use. With the transfer of these infirmaries to public health authorities, this legitimate and urgently needed use of hospital beds will further increase.

Among the chief present evils of poor law administration is that of unconditional out-door relief.

The Majority Report of the Royal Commission on Poor Laws stated: "Opinions may differ as to the degrees of strictness desirable in Poor Law administration; but no possible justification can be advanced for the granting of out-relief in such a way as to perpetuate pauperism and the evil conditions which give rise to pauperism." (Part IV, par. 261.)

In Part IV, par. 264 they added: "From the point of view of phthisis alone there is harm being done which far outweighs any benefit to be derived from the dole of out-relief. And children who are brought up in the very midst of such conditions as we have seen, surrounded by disease and immorality and drunkenness, are almost doomed to pauperism."

In paragraph 268 they stated: "We recommend that in future it should be a condition of out-relief that the recipients are leading respectable lives in decent houses."

And they forecasted that " a policy such as this " (amounting to a proscribing of dirt, and insanitary houses and areas) " gradually but steadily pursued until it was generally recognised, would, we are convinced, do much to diminish the evils of dirt, overcrowding and immorality not only amongst the actual recipients of relief, but also among their neighbours." (Part IV, par. 270.)

The present conditions as to treatment of the sick in workhouses and infirmaries vary greatly. At the time when the Royal Commission reported, in many of these institutions the hospital treatment was unskilled, no specialists were appointed for special cases, and both medical and nursing staff were inadequate. In some larger towns and in London many Poor Law Infirmaries can now rank with good general hospitals of the voluntary type. In some of them a consultant service is supplied, although often the medical and nursing staff is still inadequate to needs. Quite recently patients who are not destitute in the ordinary sense of that word are being admitted in increasing numbers to some of these institutions. Thus at the West Middlesex Hospital (Brentford Union) it is stated that about 60 per cent. of the in-patients contribute to the cost of their treatment according to their means.

Midwifery wards in these poor law hospitals are not used to anything like their capacity ; and there is little hope of improvement in this respect, until poor law medical treatment becomes part of a public health service.

The anomalous position of the Poor Law was emphasised in the National Health Insurance Act,

1911, which definitely excluded Poor Law institutions from the right to provide beds for consumptive insured persons under the Act. This action was modified, so far as concerns the Metropolitan Asylums Board (representing all the Poor Law Guardians of the metropolis); and it is now in process of being slowly broken down as regards general cases of sickness. But the position will remain unsatisfactory until medical treatment is entirely dissociated from the poor-law organisation.

Some recent improvements in poor-law administration should be noted at this point. A special Departmental Committee was appointed by Mr. John Burns to consider the recommendations of the Royal Commission on the Poor Laws relating to outdoor relief. There was issued afterwards the Relief Regulation Order, 1911, which strictly limited relief to institutional (resident) relief, except in certain cases such as sickness or accident, or bodily or mental infirmity (old age, etc.), for expenses of burial, and for widows not having illegitimate children.

The two chief forms of outdoor or domiciliary relief are monetary and medical. There is still much discussion as to the adequacy of monetary relief and the conditions which should be attached to it.

It might easily be given under conditions inimical to thrift; but there are certain safeguards against this. The main provisions are embodied in a circular of the Local Government Board of 18th March, 1910, which recommends that "when outdoor relief is given it should be carefully adapted to the needs of the case and adequate in amount." By the Outdoor Relief (Friendly Societies) Act, 1904, it was provided that in granting outdoor relief to a member of a friendly society, the Board of Guardians shall not take into consideration any sum received from such friendly society as sick pay, except any excess over 5*s.* a week. A similar provision was introduced in Sec. 109 of the National Insurance Act, 1911; and in the third schedule of the National Insurance Act, 1920, the amount 7*s.* 6*d.* was substituted for 5*s.* The Old Age Pensions Act, 1919, removed the disqualification for a pension of a person in receipt of poor law relief which had been imposed by the Old Age Pensions Act, 1908, unless where a person is receiving institutional relief for longer than three months.

For purposes of medical relief the whole of England is divided into districts, each having one or more Medical Officers appointed by the Guardians, whose duty is to attend punctually and adequately upon all poor persons requiring medical attendance, and supply any requisite medicines. He is generally underpaid for this work. Most medical officers are engaged also in general private medical practice. In most districts the call on their services, except for special certificates and for arranging the removal of patients to a poor law infirmary has declined, with the increasing amount of institutional relief, and the introduction of the Medical Benefit under the National Insurance Act.

The poor law medical officers number over 3,400, and had the recommendations of the Royal Commission on the Poor Laws been adopted, and these transferred to the larger public health authorities, there would have been immediate possibility of making them the starting point of an official medical service for insured persons, without cessation of private practice, their numbers being increased in accordance with the requirements of insurance medical practice. This has some bearing on the commonly expressed wish that some other method of payment than by capitation fee should be adopted in the National Insurance work. It would be advantageous if several methods of payment could be adopted in different localities, including the one indicated above, viz. a part-time salary.

Institutional relief is chiefly for the sick and the infirm and aged. It is hampered by the facts that

(1) The institution being intended for paupers, admission to it necessitates, except in an emergency, prior inquiry by a relieving officer, and a certification of destitution at least so far as concerns the special help which the institution can furnish.

(2) A large proportion of the Boards of Guardians have failed to classify the inmates of their institutions satisfactorily, and there is much improper mingling of different diseases and of persons who for moral or other reasons should not be associated.

Efforts have been made by the Central Ministry and by some Boards of Guardians to secure a more satisfactory classification of inmates, making treatment more economical when results obtained are considered and altogether more satisfactory. Thus imbecile, epileptic and feeble-minded persons should be removed from the general workhouse, though it does not follow that they should be transferred to lunatic asylums. Similarly advanced and active cases of tuberculosis should always be treated in special wards; as also should all cases of venereal diseases. In the metropolis and some large towns this is already done; but there is need for further differentiation which probably will only be secured in the metropolis, for instance, when, for this purpose, London becomes a single authority. For certain diseases this has already been secured by the Metropolitan Asylums Board. This body illustrates the transition from poor law to public health; for although it is technically a poor law authority it performs mainly public health functions. It is formed chiefly from representatives sent by the different Metropolitan Boards of Guardians, and is thus not a popularly elected body. It provides excellent institutional treatment for acute infectious diseases, for tuberculosis, for the feeble-minded, and for various other diseases; and, although a Poor Law organisation, it is forbidden to recover payment for the treatment of fever and smallpox patients who are not destitute.

Excepting the Metropolitan Asylums Board and a few other authorities, two great defects, now in too slow process of improvement, have characterised institutional relief under the Poor Law: (1) inadequate medical staff, without consultant facilities, (2) unsatisfactory nursing. The Poor Law Institutions (Nursing) Order, 1913, prohibits the employment of any inmate for nursing the sick, and prohibits also the employment of an inmate in any capacity in the sick wards, the lunatic wards, or the nurseries, unless approved by the Medical Officer for this particular work and acting under the immediate supervision of a paid officer.

It is essential that the workhouse or general institution should be entirely separate in administration from the administration of the sick wards, and this is the increasing policy of progressive Boards of Guardians. Were their duties exercised by them as largely autonomous Committees of the County or County Borough Council, there is little doubt that this rule would become general; and that the utility of these hospitals would be enormously increased by their becoming the headquarters for various public health, school, and insurance clinics, and by their supplying greatly needed beds for non-poor law tuberculosis, venereal disease, maternity and other cases.

For children under the Poor Law much has been done. Some provision has always been needed for orphans or deserted children, or children who for some other reason cannot be supported by their parents. In the past they have been unsatisfactorily left in workhouses; but by the Poor Law Institutions Order, 1913, of the Local Government Board, healthy boys and girls, aged 3 to 16, were not allowed to be retained in institutions for adults for a period exceeding six weeks, unless under a medical certificate. This Order is not completely enforced. The various schemes of dealing with children, as in poor law schools, by boarding out, in cottage and scattered homes, etc. can only be mentioned.

The general considerations as to medical assistance to the public will be better stated after medical treatment under the National Insurance Act and the medical treatment of school children have been described.

Chapter XIV

HEALTH INSURANCE AND THE PUBLIC HEALTH

To understand the position of National Insurance against sickness, the circumstances and time of its initiation need to be remembered. In 1908 Mr. Asquith, as Chancellor of the Exchequer, introduced the Old Age Pensions Act, which provided a weekly pension of 5*s.* to every person over 70 years of age, who for ten years prior to reaching this age had been a British subject. This has been amended by more recent Acts in 1911, 1920, and 1924, the weekly amount being increased to 10*s.* Under the former Acts if the applicant had an income from private sources of more than 10*s.* a week the pension was proportionately reduced. The new Act of 1924 lays down that income up to 15*s.* a week from any other source except earnings will not be counted in estimating the amount of income.

The Blind Persons Act, 1920, reduces the statutory age for the receipt of an old age pension from 70 to 50, for persons who are so blind as to be unable to perform work for which eyesight is essential.

It will be noted that the pensions were not made dependent on contributions in earlier life; and some objection has been raised on this point. A large proportion of the beneficiaries, were it not for the pension would be costing the community a larger sum as inmates of workhouses and infirmaries; though in practice many pensioners are obliged to resort to these institutions when sick or infirm, in order to receive adequate attention.

In 1909 the Poor Law Commission, which had been sitting for four years, issued its two reports, a majority report signed by fourteen, and a minority report by four Commissioners.

The two reports made valuable recommendations in common, among which the following may be briefly indicated.

(1) It was agreed that *Boards of Guardians should be abolished*, and that the area of administration should be enlarged from the Union to the county and county borough (page 145).

This conclusion arose out of the urgent necessity for

(2) The *abolition of the general mixed workhouse* and the substitution of classified institutions. The Commissioners drew attention to the fact that although the evils of general mixed workhouses were realised in 1834, they persisted in the institutions of to-day.

(3) In view of the important relation between charity and the relief of distress, the Commissioners proposed a scheme of *organisation of voluntary aid.*

(4) They urged the *removal of all children from workhouses.*

(5) They laid down rules for *improved administration of outdoor relief*, including recommendations for full inquiry, for adequacy to needs, and for supervision of the persons relieved, especially as to the moral and sanitary conditions under which they live.

Some of these recommendations have already been partially adopted.

The majority report recommended that a Committee of the county council or county borough council should be appointed for the giving of Public Assistance, one-half of whose members should consist of members of the council and one half of persons from outside their number; while the minority report favoured the relegation of care of the non-able-bodied necessitous to the Education Committee for children of school age; to the Health Committee for sick and infants; to the Asylums Committee for mentally defective, etc.

As already stated (page 145) the two reports have been reconsidered, and the adjustment set out on page 146 has been arranged.

The existence of these two reports gave a feeble excuse for the inauguration of a national system of insurance against sickness, which ignored existing official conditions and arrangements. This decision was deplorable. The two reports of the Royal Commission on the Poor Laws embodied an urgent body of needed reform, on which there was agreement. Reform of local governing areas as well as of the poor law organisation was admittedly required; and, although difficult, this would have redounded and will still redound greatly to the credit of those daring to tackle it. Instead of this the National (Health) Insurance Bill was introduced in 1911, which necessarily ran athwart the needed course of development and reform in public health administration.

In considering this problem it is necessary to bear

in mind some considerations bearing on the *relation of sickness to the prevention of sickness.*

The long and honourable history of the chief Friendly Societies of this country, who have organised a system of contributions during health, in order to be able to give money benefits and medical attendance during sickness and burial grant in the event of death, shows that in this country there has been a widespread appreciation of the need for co-operative insurance against certain contingencies of life. Individual health and life are uncertain, but in the aggregate the average incidence of sickness and mortality can be forecast; and insurance through Friendly Societies or otherwise forms an admirable method for the *collective bearing of risks*, which to the individual would be an intolerable burden.

Insurance against sickness, however, assumes the necessary continuance of sickness; and *per se* such insurance makes no provision for the reduction of sickness. In other words insurance is not prevention. It would, for instance, be ridiculous to insure against smallpox, for which vaccination supplies a complete personal protection. Even for such diseases as typhoid fever or diphtheria, against which known and effective preventive measures are practicable, insurance is inappropriate, unless one is obliged to live in places where these diseases prevail to excess or preventive measures cannot immediately be utilised.

Insurance is not an alternative to prevention, but if satisfactorily organised it may facilitate and stimulate preventive measures. To this end the persons insured must be led to interest themselves in the preventive problem. When they realise that additional benefits can be secured by reduction of the claims insurance will go hand in hand with prevention. Fire insurances or motor accident insurances illustrate this point. It may pay the insurance society to send agents to inspect premises or cars to ascertain that preventive measures are being carried out; and the same end is sought by the reduction of annual premiums if no accident occurs. A chief objection to insurance among the various societies now operating under the National Insurance Act is the high cost of weekly collection of funds, which may be one-fifth of the total amount contributed. It must be admitted furthermore that in the State system, especially in the newer Societies not on the old Friendly Society basis, the old comradeship and sense of collective responsibility have been lost.

But notwithstanding these and other drawbacks, the various forms of Social Insurance now in force are doing excellent work. They all strike more or less successfully at one of the greatest evils in life—*uncertainty of continuous ability to maintain self and family*. This is the nightmare which must haunt the minds of intelligent wage-earners. It is a cause of mental distress and anxiety, and is therefore inimical to health, only less so than accident or unemployment or sickness—the three chief causes of anxiety in operation before old age creeps on—when no prior provision has been made. In view of the importance to health of removal or reduction of this haunting uncertainty a précis is given here of the chief State provisions so far made.

Compensation for Injuries.—This was begun in 1897, and extended in 1906 to almost every industry. It now includes certain defined industrial diseases as well as accidents. The benefit for total incapacity is half wages with a maximum of 30*s.* a week; there are other benefits for partial incapacity and for dependents in case of fatal accidents.

Old Age Pensions.—These were begun in 1908. No contribution has been paid by the pensioner, except in so far as he has contributed to national expenditure during his past life. In the wider sense of the word this may be regarded as a form of insurance. See also page 184.

Unemployment Insurance.—Labour Exchanges were initiated in 1909, and a compulsory system of insurance against unemployment was adopted for a limited number of industries in Part II of the National Health Insurance Act, 1911. In later Acts in 1916 and 1920 the scope of the scheme was extended; and it now applies to all persons included in sickness insurance except out-workers, or agricultural employees, or persons in domestic service. It applies to about 12 million persons as compared with 15 millions for health insurance. At first for men 4*d.* was the weekly contribution of employer and of employed person. The unprecedented amount of unemployment in recent years necessitated amending Acts and in 1921 the weekly contribution of the employer was increased to 10*d.*, and of the employed man aged 18 or over to 9*d.*, making a total of 1*s.* 7*d.*, to which the State contributes rather more than one-third of the joint contribution. The benefits have been 18*s.* per week for men and

15*s*. for women, with an additional benefit of 5*s*. for wives, and 2*s*. for each child of married men.

Sickness and Disablement.—Insurance against sickness and disablement for wage-earners (all persons over 16) and other employees as defined in the National Health Insurance Act, 1924, was initiated by the Act of 1911, as was also Unemployment Insurance.

For the employers of men and the employed the weekly payment required is 5*d*. each; for women employed the payment is 4*d*., the employer paying 5*d*. These together form seven-ninths of the contributions, the remaining two-ninths being supplied from moneys provided by Parliament.

Sickness Insurance Benefits.—There are now four ordinary benefits under the National (Health) Insurance Act, viz.,

(1) Medical Benefit.
(2) Cash Benefits.
(*a*) For sickness.
(*b*) For disablement.
(*c*) For maternity.

After a probationary period the normal sickness benefit for a man is 15*s*., for a woman 12*s*. a week throughout an entire twenty-six weeks, and both alike are subsequently entitled to disablement benefit of 7*s*. 6*d*. a week for so long as disablement continues up to the age of 70.

Maternity Benefit is 40*s*. for the wife of an insured man, or double this amount if she also is an employed person under the terms of the Act. It is doubtful whether this is the best form that this benefit could take. Free attendance by a doctor and midwife supplemented by the provision of domestic help during the lying-in period, or free attendance in a Maternity Home would be more certainly beneficial to both mother and infant than the present monetary grant, or a grant which would be partially monetary and partially in direct service. It would be in the public interest if the administration of the Maternity Benefit were transferred from the Approved Societies to the larger public health authorities, as in the case of the Sanatorium Benefit; but the two cases differ in that the funds for the Maternity Benefit are derived from the Society's funds; and to effect the change it will apparently be necessary to nationalise the funds of all Friendly Societies. But the transfer is most desirable, the administration of this Benefit on better lines fitting in closely with existent maternity and child welfare work of public health authorities.

Medical Benefit entitles to medical attendance and treatment, including such medical and surgical appliances as may be prescribed by regulations. It does not include specialist or dental treatment, unless the Society to which the insured person belongs gives additional benefits. It includes ordinary attendance on cases of tuberculosis; but the former Sanatorium Benefit has been abandoned, as public health authorities give institutional treatment for tuberculosis, whether insured or non-insured. It does not include attendance in confinement for insured women, the maternity benefit in cash taking the place of this.

Although sickness insurance has not, as at present organised, a marked influence in the prevention of disease, it can be claimed for it that it provides without let or hindrance access to a qualified medical practitioner of the patient's own choice for any illness however slight; and this opens out the possibility of early and of uninterrupted and continued treatment of sickness, which ought to diminish its severity and its duration. If sickness is thus handled, disease becomes less serious and its disabling complications rare. There should be no insuperable difficulty in attaining to this point and in advancing beyond it; for the arrangements with panel doctors might be extended to include the duty on the part of each doctor of making himself acquainted with the domestic, social, and industrial life of his patient, giving him advice on any unhygienic habits or conditions, and when this appeared desirable overhauling his potential patient by a physical examination. Legally this extension of the doctor's work may be regarded as coming almost within the terms of his present contract; and it may be argued further that not only does this proposal introduce the doctor into the sphere of preventive medicine—his ideal sphere—but that his work in this direction should diminish his own therapeutic work, as well as the drain on insurance funds for sick benefit.

It is furthermore true that illness at an early stage, when a careful medical examination and diagnosis is made, may be so treated as to constitute a valuable part of preventive medicine (see page 259). Prevention of death and prevention or reduction of invalidity though not so important as prevention of disease have great national and personal value.

Even at the present time many panel doctors are giving therapeutic services to their patients which could not be improved. Often this is not so; either the doctor has too many patients, or he differentiates between private and panel patients, or he fails to realise the importance of an expert consultation, or of hospital treatment, or of skilled nursing for his patient, and he fails to secure these. These last named failures are not surprising, because most of the Societies through whom the Act is administered have not the special benefits required for difficult cases.

The essential defect of the Medical Benefit is that while it furnishes medical attendance for minor ailments and for such more serious illnesses as come within the ordinary average competence of a medical practitioner, there is no provision, unless the insured person happens to belong to a Society having surplus funds, for such specialist services as

(1) Consultation with experts in various branches of medicine and surgery (except gratuitously at hospitals, or occasionally through the Divisional Medical Officers of the Ministry of Health);

(2) Hospital treatment, as in operation cases, or in cases where home circumstances are inimical to recovery, except gratuitously;

(3) Dental treatment;

(4) Skilled nursing.

The services of the Public Health Authority are available for cases of tuberculosis and of venereal disease where expert treatment is required; for some acute infectious diseases; and possibly for special cases of sickness during the pregnancy of an insured person.

From the preceding outline of the well known facts bearing on Social Insurance we may, I think, form the following conclusions :—

(1) Insurance itself is not a means of preventing the evil against which one insures ; but it may be made a handmaid of prevention.

(2) Unless redoubled efforts are taken to reduce the evils insured against, insurance may even do harm morally and socially.

(3) The one form of insurance to which these potential objections against insurance apply least of all, is the giving of old age pensions, whether on a contributory basis, or as at present out of national funds to which all contribute.

(4) Insurance against unemployment is a necessary implement in our social armamentarium, and like sickness insurance it is now in force for nearly one-third of the total population, and for a much higher proportion of the adult population. As in the case of the other forms of insurance, it does not prevent unemployment, and makes it all the more necessary to search out the causes of unemployment and so to regulate unemployment insurance that it may not be abused.

(5) Insurance against sickness can be made to conduce to recovery by diminishing financial anxiety, by supplying some of the familiar means conducing to recovery, and by rendering possible early and continuous treatment of sickness to the extent to which this treatment is skilful and appropriate to special needs.

Such insurance holds within it the possibility of preventing a large amount of sickness, if the doctor selected by the patient is utilised for preventive advice as well as for curative treatment.

(6) The possibilities of good of the maternity benefit might be greatly increased, if its organisation were revised, as recommended on page 191.

Chapter XV

ADMINISTRATION OF HEALTH INSURANCE AND THE PUBLIC HEALTH

THE methods of administration of the national system of sickness insurance have important bearings on public health administration, both central and local. In reading the National Health Insurance Act, 1924, which consolidates the original Act of 1911 and several intermediate modifying Acts, it would appear that the Central Government's duties are not very extensive; but in fact administrative regulation is very centralised. As already seen (page 126) the central work of the National Insurance Act is now carried out in a special division of the Ministry of Health. This work includes the approval of Societies, the making of Regulations, action through specially appointed Commissioners as a Court of Appeal for Societies, and so on. The chief work of insurance was intended to be done by two bodies, viz. Approved Societies and Insurance Committees.

The Approved Societies constitute the essential part of the machinery of the scheme. To them is entrusted the task of administering the three cash benefits of the Act (sickness, disablement, and maternity), and in doing this they enjoy almost complete autonomy. Medical practitioners, when the Insurance Bill of 1911 was before Parliament, announced that they would not serve under Approved Societies; and this was not surprising in view of the unsatisfactory conditions of Club practice of the past under Friendly Society administration. It was necessary therefore to create a separate Committee to deal with medical benefits. This was done by the appointment of an Insurance Committee in every county and county borough, which arranges for the inclusion of every doctor desiring it to be placed on the local "Medical List," thus rendering him available for choice by insured persons.

The constitution of these two bodies should be noted. The Approved Society must not be a Society carried on for profit; and "its constitution must provide to the satisfaction of the Minister (of Health) for its affairs being subject to the absolute control of its members being insured persons or, if the rules of the society so provide, of its members whether insured persons or not."

The Insurance Committee may consist of twenty to forty members of whom (*a*) three-fifths shall be appointed so as to secure representation of the insured persons in the county or county borough; (*b*) one-fifth shall be appointed by the council of the county or county borough; (*c*) two members shall be appointed by a local medical committee for the area; (*d*) one shall be a medical practitioner appointed by the local council; and (*e*) the remaining members shall be appointed by the Minister. At least four members of this Committee are required to be women.

Evidently there is ample provision for autonomy

on the part of the Approved Societies; but in actual fact the work of the Societies has fallen almost entirely into the hands of paid officials, and there is an unfortunate absence of the interest in local insurance administration which characterised insured persons under the old Friendly Societies having local branches. This is not surprising in view of the fact that the members of the Society are now much more delocalised than in the past—may be scattered throughout the entire country. A further reason is that this class of insurance work has been taken up by Industrial Insurance Companies and by Trades Unions, to which it is somewhat of a "side show." Whatever the reasons, the old Friendly Society management with its sense of corporate responsibility has become exceptional, and with it one of the chief reasons—on the merits—for the retention of approved non-national societies for insurance has disappeared.

There is a further weakness in the position of Approved Societies. They can recruit their members from a particular occupation or place, or from miscellaneous sources. Each Society can admit or reject any person applying for membership, provided that the rejection shall not be solely on the ground of the age of the applicant. There has resulted a gradual stratification or segregation of insured persons, societies having members with an excessive proportion of very healthy or of very sickly persons. Hence on a large scale we have "sectional insurance not national insurance, the strong bearing the burdens of the strong, and the weak the burdens of the weak." Thus domestic servants, who have little sickness and often do not claim benefits to which they are entitled, tend to collect in special societies; while other societies, e.g. in mining or densely populated districts have members with a high rate of sickness. This may be regarded as a necessary difference between insurance and taxation; but when, as in this case, the State and employers contribute together more largely than the insured, the argument for spreading out risks to the utmost and for preventing "sectionalisation" of the insured funds becomes unanswerable.

Associated with this fundamentally erroneous sectional distribution of insurance, a miner or a dock labourer pays no higher contribution than an agricultural labourer though the incidence of sickness is very excessive in the former.

To put this right, national pooling of payments and equalised distribution of benefits would be required, which may not at present be practicable.

The work of the Insurance Committee need not be further particularised. Reference may be made to the general observations on page 191. About half the medical practitioners in the country accept insurance patients, payment being arranged in most areas on the basis of a capitation payment of 9*s*. per annum for each person on the doctor's list. This number averages about 1,000, and a doctor may not have on his list more than 2,500 insured persons. The disciplinary part of the work of this Committee sometimes involves reporting an individual doctor to the Ministry of Health, whose quasi-judicial functions have already been mentioned (page 85).

Sec. 107 of the Act of 1924 (Sec. 60 of that of 1911) gives power to any approved society or insurance committee to make representations to any person or authority that in their opinion the sickness among insured persons is excessive owing to (*a*) conditions of employment, (*b*) bad housing or insanitary conditions, (*c*) contaminated water supply, (*d*) neglect of provisions of any Act relating to industrial or housing conditions, for which such person or authority is alleged by them to be responsible; and the Minister of Health may order an inquiry in such a case, if he holds that a *primâ facie* case has been made out.

So far as I know, action has never been taken under this clause. It was an ill-conceived procedure, arising possibly out of a failure to appreciate that the organisation of Approved Societies could not give the local distribution of sickness among their members.

Under Sec. 50 of the Act of 1924 the duty is imposed on the local Insurance Committee of "making such reports as to the health of insured persons . . . as the Minister may prescribe," and of arranging to give lectures and publish information on questions relating to health if they think this necessary or desirable. The medical officer of health may be called in to advise the Insurance Committee, but he has no statutory relation to the Committee, nor has the Committee any statutory relation to the local public health authorities (County Council or County Borough Council), unless the one-fifth representation of these bodies on the Insurance Committee gives a simulacrum of this.

Some further medical assistance is now possible by the appointment of thirty-six Medical Referees by the Ministry of Health who will be able to help medical practitioners in difficult cases in which a second medical opinion is desired, and especially where malingering is suspected, while supplying a useful check in cases of careless certification of sickness. There is little hope of much useful statistical investigation of the health of insured persons until certification is more accurate, and until it becomes possible to obtain adequate evidence on a geographical or an occupational basis, which appears rarely practicable with the present arrangement of societies. I may sum up by quoting from a recent address given by me to the Poor Law Medical Association :—

> "The difficulties of insurance relate among other things to the excessive cost of the system, due to the present conditions of administration ; to the constant tendency towards the 'segregation of good lives' ; to the infrequency of geographical distribution of the insured in societies ; and to the non-correspondence between the monetary allowance in sickness and the duration of the need for this.
>
> "The struggling and the sick in the societies in which they are most numerous need most and get least, which is contrary to the spirit of all public health work : inordinate and extravagant book-keeping and correspondence are involved in the present non-geographical distribution of members in societies ; and chaos of insurance administration is ensured by the fact that insurance

committees are local, while societies of insured are not similarly localised, and the further fact that insurance committees are not organically related to public health authorities.

"On the medical side, is insurance, as now organised, a hand-maiden of public health? It is a safe proposition that although insurance in itself is a valuable provision for contingencies, it is harmful to the extent to which it conduces to contentment with the *status quo* and fails to provide means for diminishing the evils insured against. The Workmen's Compensation Act is open to a similar objection. In itself it has little or no influence in reducing the number of accidents; and in this essential respect the administration of the Factory and Mines Departments of the Home Office stands on a much higher platform. In America, and to some extent here this antithesis is being recognised; and the extensive issue at the expense of insurance societies of pamphlets and notices on 'Safety First' represents valuable social work as well as sound business instincts. Let us not forget, however, that unless carefully safeguarded, insurance against sickness, like Poor Law work, will not diminish the evils relieved.

"Our present national system of insurance against sickness is hitherto a most imperfect instrument even for the treatment of disease. The great majority of cases medically treated by the doctor in his contract are slight in character; and voluntary and Poor Law and public health hospitals provide for a high proportion of the total serious cases. There is extremely inadequate provision for medical consultations in difficult cases, for the treatment of various diseases needing the skill of the specialist, for skilled nursing, and for dental treatment. Above all, there is little provision out of insurance funds for hospital treatment of thousands of patients who, without it, cannot be successfully treated."

Criticism is fairly easy; and it is necessary to supplement it by constructive suggestions, assuming that the changes needed to secure sound and economical insurance administration will be faced. The ideal undoubtedly would be to nationalise the health insurance service, as the unemployment and pensions services have been nationalised. In the case of health insurance localised health functions are needed, and it would be desirable to have county or county borough administration through an almost completely autonomous insurance committee formed by representatives of the medical profession, of insured persons and of the local authority. By this means the general sickness experience of one-third of the total population could be brought under review by the medical officer of health, or of an expert hygienist in his department, and early inquiries into preventable or controllable illness could be made. Insurance work would take its place side by side with other forms of health work as it does centrally at the Ministry of Health.

The present Insurance Committees, owing to the centralisation of their work by means of the

Ministry of Health's regulations, have almost nothing to do; and they cannot be revitalised except by reception into the Local Public Health Authority.

Chapter XVI

THE MINISTRATION OF HEALTH FOR CHILDREN

THE general scope of central and public health administration will have been gathered from the preceding chapters, and is seen in a summarised form in the statements on pages 96, 44—48. In view of their importance in the evolution of health administration, some special statement appears to be required in regard to children under school age (0-5), and for two diseases, viz. tuberculosis and venereal disease (comprising syphilis and gonorrhœa), to which special administrative measures have been directed.

These three new public health services were initiated as separate divisions of public health work, with the stimulus of grants-in-aid, during the last ten years of the Local Government Board's existence.

The child has been a chief motive in social improvement during the last hundred years and longer; and it is by increased legislative control and by the concurrent force of public opinion, becoming more and more educated, that much of the progress secured has been rendered possible.

For the infant, as for the aged in the last stage of life, tenure of life is slender, and the line of demarcation between physiological order and disorder, between health and sickness, may almost daily be passed. Since Budin in 1892 first inaugurated his infant consultations in Paris, immense progress has been made in the treatment and still more in the prevention of infantile ailments. Knowledge has spread to an extent which puts the poorest mother of to-day in a better position to secure her infant's health than were the well-to-do a generation ago. There is no department of medicine in which prevention has superseded treatment to the extent which holds good for infants. The average mother knows the need of orange juice for her infant, when the substitution of artificial feeding for mother's milk is unavoidable; and she is ready to administer cod liver oil to prevent infantile rickets, even without medical advice. She is rapidly learning also the value of exposure of the infant to sunshine. The result is that infantile scurvy is rarely seen, and rickets in its fully developed form has become a relatively rare instead of a common disease.

Unfortunately one cannot say that after infancy improved hygiene holds sway to the same extent. At ages between 2 and 5 there has been a marvellous reduction of tuberculosis and of acute infectious diseases; but at these ages the child's health is not adequately supervised, and dental decay, adenoids, tonsillar infections, and disturbances of behaviour which might have been corrected earlier, are commonly found when the child enters school. That the condition of the child will improve at these ages as much as it has already done in infancy, may be expected as child welfare work and the enlightenment of mothers progresses.

The influence of a growing national sensitiveness to the wrongs of children on the development of state control has been pre-eminently great. The first interference with complete license to exploit workers was in regard to children employed to sweep chimneys. The interference with so-called freedom of contract soon extended to children employed in factories, and ere long included compulsion to supply a modicum of education to such children (page 5).

The importance already attached to child welfare is strikingly illustrated by the Children Act, 1908, containing 134 clauses in six parts dealing with Infant Life Protection, Prevention of Cruelty to Children and Young Persons, Juvenile Smoking, and Reformatory and Industrial Schools, Juvenile Offenders, and other miscellaneous matters.

On the public health side, one of the earliest statistical investigations of the Privy Council was into the causation of Epidemic Diarrhœa, a disease especially fatal to infants. Similar investigations into this and other causes of excessive infantile mortality have followed on the part of many medical officers of health. Early in the present century the appointment of female health visitors became not uncommon, although I noted in my Annual Report to the Local Government Board for 1909-10, that doubt had been raised as to the legal powers of a Sanitary Authority to pay their salaries, and that to clear up the doubt the London County Council had obtained special Parliamentary powers for this purpose.

Efforts for the control of infant mortality were

greatly increased during Mr. John Burns' presidency of the Local Government Board, and the policy of "concentration on the mother and her child" began to show result in rapid reduction of infant mortality.

The Notification of Births Act, passed in 1907, and made obligatory in all areas in 1915, greatly increased the possibilities of child welfare work. The birth of each infant was required to be notified to the medical officer of health within thirty-six hours of its birth; and in this way it became possible to make early and repeated visits to the parent, for the giving of counsel on the health of the mother and her child.

Reference may also be made to a series of reports on infant and child mortality, and on maternal mortality issued from the Medical Department of the Local Government Board during the same period. These efforts culminated in the issue on the 30th July, 1914, of a circular which in view of its national importance is here reproduced. It had been carefully prepared; and fortunately the almost immediately subsequent announcement of war was not allowed to inhibit child welfare work.

During the war this work still further advanced. The 50 per cent. Treasury Grants then promised made progress easier; although confusion and overlapping of work arose owing to the Board of Education having obtained consent also to give grants in respect of "schools for mothers" and allied work. These were practically indistinguishable from the "infant consultations" and associated work which were being subsidised by the Local

Government Board. This confusion disappeared when the Ministry of Health Act came into force.

Circular.
County Councils
and
Sanitary Authorities.

LOCAL GOVERNMENT BOARD,
Whitehall, S.W.
30th July, 1914.

MATERNITY AND CHILD WELFARE

SIR,

I am directed by the Local Government Board to state that an estimate has been laid before Parliament for a grant to be distributed by the Board in aid of the expenditure of local authorities and voluntary agencies in respect of institutions or other provision for maternity and child welfare.

This grant, if voted by Parliament, will be made in aid of expenditure in respect of clinics, dispensaries or other institutions primarily concerned with the provision of medical and surgical advice and treatment, as well as in respect of the salaries of health visitors and other officers engaged for this work.

The Local Government Board have in recent years devoted considerable attention to questions connected with infant welfare and they have observed with much satisfaction that efforts have been made by many local authorities and voluntary agencies, to deal with the matter. These efforts have undoubtedly helped to secure improved conditions for children and have played an important part in the campaign for the reduction of infantile mortality.

It is evident from the Reports issued by the Medical Department of the Board and those of many Medical Officers of Health that more extended and systematic measures than have hitherto been generally adopted are necessary, and it is hoped that the grant of assistance from the Exchequer will stimulate those local authorities who have not yet taken action to give the matter their earnest consideration and will encourage those already engaged in work to develop it still further.

Up to the present local authorities, in their infant welfare work, have concerned themselves more especially with the child in its first year of life; the matter is, however, one which needs to be dealt with on a more comprehensive basis and it is clearly desirable that there should be continuity in dealing with the whole period from before birth until the time when the child is entered upon a school register, i.e. the register of a public elementary school, nursery school, crèche, day nursery, school for mothers, or other school.

Extension of the existing work is accordingly needed in two directions; on the one hand it is necessary that measures should be taken for securing improved ante-natal and natal conditions, and on the other, provision should be made for continuing the work in relation to children beyond the first year of life.

The accompanying memorandum, which has been prepared by the Board's Medical Officer with a view to assisting the formulation of schemes or extending the work already undertaken, sets forth in outline the matters needing consideration in the preparation of a comprehensive scheme. It will be seen that the memorandum contemplates that medical advice and, where necessary, treatment should be continuously and systematically available for expectant mothers and for children till they are entered on a school register, and that arrangements should be made for home visitation throughout this period.

The work of home visitation is one to which the Board attach very great importance, and in promoting schemes on the lines laid down in the accompanying statement the first step should be the appointment of an adequate staff of Health Visitors.

It will be desirable, at all events in the case of the larger urban authorities, to provide consultation centres which may fitly be termed Maternity Centres, to which expectant mothers and mothers with infants and little children may be referred for advice and treatment; the operation of these Maternity Centres will be rendered most effective if co-operation is secured with the midwives of the district and with any local hospital having a maternity department.

It will be necessary to arrange for a medical officer to be in charge of such a Centre and for the attendance at the Centre of members of the staff engaged in home visiting. Careful records, for which the medical officer should be responsible, will need to be kept, and in regard to children the records should be in such a form that they may subsequently be available for the information of the School Medical Officer when the child is entered at a school.

For the rural and smaller urban areas the Board think it will generally be found desirable to develop a county organisation, but in all cases the county work should be intimately related with that of the local sanitary authority, and on the other hand any work separately undertaken by a sanitary authority should be co-ordinated with the county scheme.

It is not expected that all local authorities will be able at once to initiate complete schemes, but it is important that any partial arrangements that may be made shall be such as can ultimately form part of a more extended organisation.

Subject to the estimate now before Parliament being accepted by Parliament, the Board will be willing to consider applications for grants in respect of any work falling within the scope of the scheme outlined in the memorandum accompanying this letter ; the grants will normally amount to one-half the approved expenditure on any of these purposes, but may be less if the Board so decide.

Grants to institutions of the nature of Schools for Mothers, the object of which is primarily educational, which provide training and instruction for mothers in the care and management of infants and little children, and which may include systematic classes, or home visiting, or infant consultations (the provision of specific medical and surgical advice and treatment, if any, being only incidental), will be administered by the Board of Education. Any cases of doubt or difficulty will be investigated by a Joint Committee of Officers of the two Boards, which will include women Medical Officers.

In sending a copy of this circular to voluntary agencies engaged in infant welfare work, the Board will state that applications for grants in respect of voluntary work may be made by a voluntary agency either directly or through a local authority.

The grant now presented to Parliament will be appropriated in aid of the expenditure of the half-year ended 30th September, 1914, and applications for grants should be accompanied by an account of the work undertaken by the authority, and by a detailed statement of the expenditure incurred, certified by the officer of the local authority in charge of the accounts.

I am to add that the Board will be happy to afford advice and assistance to local authorities in the initiation of schemes or the extension of existing schemes.

I am, Sir, Your obedient servant,

The Clerk to the Council. H. C. Monro, Secretary.

MATERNITY AND CHILD WELFARE.

A complete scheme would comprise the following elements, each of which will, in this connection, be organised in its direct bearing on infantile health.

1. Arrangements for the local supervision of Midwives.

2. Arrangements for—

ANTE-NATAL.
(1) An ante-natal clinic for expectant mothers.
(2) The home visiting of expectant mothers.
(3) A maternity hospital or beds at a hospital, in which complicated cases of pregnancy can receive treatment.

3. Arrangements for—

NATAL.
(1) Such assistance as may be needed to ensure the mother having skilled and prompt attendance during confinement at home.
(2) The confinement of sick women, including women having contracted pelvis or suffering from any other condition involving danger to the mother or infant, at a hospital.

4. Arrangements for—

POST-NATAL.
(1) The treatment in a hospital of complications arising after parturition, whether in the mother or in the infant.
(2) The provision of systematic advice and treatment for infants at a baby clinic or infant dispensary.
(3) The continuance of these clinics and dispensaries, so as to be available for children up to the age when they are entered on a school register, i.e. the register of a public elementary school, nursery school, crèche, day nursery, school for mothers or other school.
(4) The systematic home visitation of infants and of children not on a school register as above defined.

LOCAL GOVERNMENT BOARD,
Whitehall, S.W.
July, 1914.

In August, 1918, a circular was issued by the Local Government Board giving more detailed particulars as to objects for which the Board were prepared to give grants not exceeding 50 per cent. of the approved expenditure.

REGULATIONS under which grants not exceeding one-half of approved net expenditure will be payable by the Local Government Board to Local Authorities and to Voluntary Agencies in respect of arrangements for attending to the health of expectant mothers and nursing mothers and of children under five years of age.

1. The Local Government Board will pay grants during each financial year, commencing on 1st April, in respect of the following services:—

(1) The salaries and expenses of Inspectors of Midwives.

(2) The salaries and expenses of Health Visitors and Nurses engaged in Maternity and Child Welfare work.

(3) The provision of a midwife for necessitous women in confinement and for areas which are insufficiently supplied with this service.

(4) The provision, for necessitous women, of a doctor for illness connected with pregnancy and for aid during the period of confinement for mother and child.

(5) The expenses of a Centre, i.e. an institution providing any or all of the following activities:—medical supervision and advice for expectant and nursing mothers, and for children under five years of age, and medical treatment at the Centre for cases needing it.

(6) Arrangements for instruction in the general hygiene of maternity and childhood.

(7) Hospital treatment provided or contracted for by Local Authorities for complicated cases of confinement or complications arising after parturition, or for cases in which a woman to be confined suffers from illness or deformity, or for cases of women who, in the opinion of the Medical Officer of Health, cannot with safety be confined in their homes or such other provision for securing proper conditions for the confinement of necessitous women as may be approved by the Medical Officer of Health.

(8) Hospital treatment provided or contracted for by Local Authorities for children under five years of age found to need in-patient treatment.

(9) The cost of food provided for expectant mothers and nursing mothers and for children under five years of age, where such provision is certified by the Medical Officer of the Centre or by the Medical Officer of Health to be necessary and where the case is necessitous.

(10) Expenses of crèches and day nurseries and of other arrangements for attending to the health of children under five years of age whose mothers go out to work.

(11) The provision of accommodation in convalescent homes for nursing mothers and for children under five years of age.

(12) The provision of homes and other arrangements for attending to the health of children of widowed, deserted and unmarried mothers, under five years of age.

(13) Experimental work for the health of expectant and nursing mothers and of infants and children under five years of age carried out by Local Authorities or voluntary agencies with the approval of the Board.

(14) Contributions by the Local Authority to voluntary institutions and agencies approved under the scheme.

2. Grants will be paid to voluntary agencies aided by the Board on condition:—

(1) That the work of the agency is approved by the Board and co-ordinated as far as practicable with the public health work of the Local Authority and the school medical service of the local education authority.

(2) That the premises and work of the institution are subject to inspection by any of the Board's Officers or Inspectors.

(3) That records of the work done by the agency are kept to the satisfaction of the Board.

During the temporary undiscriminating restriction of expenditure after the Great War, these grants were seriously restricted, but have since then been restored, and the amount of money thus expended by the Exchequer during 1922-3 is stated on page 110.

The ideals of this work are to improve the health of the expectant mother and to safeguard her against the dangers of childbearing; to ensure for the infant the initial good start which parental health and efficiency and breast feeding can promote; to protect the infant against the dietetic and other hygienic dangers of infancy; and to continue this protection during the next four years of life when the child is assumed to come within the range of school medical inspection. In carrying out this work medical observation and occasional examination of children are rendered of much greater value by the visits of health visitors to the home of the child; and this home visitation is almost the most important element in the whole work.

The number of health visitors in April, 1924, in England and Wales was 3,635, of whom 888 were employed wholly in maternity and child welfare; 1,129 acted also as school nurse, tuberculosis nurse, or sanitary inspector; and 1,276 were district nurses employed by voluntary nursing associations, who were employed by county councils for health visiting in rural areas. The desirability of such combined duties depends upon geographical and other considerations. In densely populated towns the balance lies perhaps in favour of health visitors devoted only to maternity and child welfare work; though if a health visitor possesses adequate practical knowledge of the work of a school nurse and of tuberculosis, it is sometimes desirable to employ her in all three capacities. This is especially so in sparsely populated areas. The combination of the work of health visiting with district nursing is less free from objection, owing to the varying demands on the time of the nurse for actual nursing. Many district nurses also have not had adequate hygienic training.

When the work of health visitors was first made the subject of central monetary grants, it was required that the health visitor should have received the full training of a nurse, or have the certificate of the Central Midwives Board, or have received a certificate of competency in health visiting from an approved society along with some training in nursing. The majority of health visitors will soon be completely trained nurses who have had special training in the duties of a health visitor.

If a health visitor devotes her whole time to maternity and child welfare work, there should be one to every 350 or 400 births in the area in which she works. This enables her to pay several visits during the first year of the infant's life, and places her in a favourable position for keeping in touch with him during the next two years of his life. Her duty is largely educational and hygienic. It must be so in part by demonstration of the best methods of feeding and dressing, and of domestic hygiene. It is largely through her influence that attendance at ante-natal and infant welfare centres is secured, thus bringing to bear medical skill on the care of mother and child. The increased knowledge of child hygiene and its wider application in the community are ascribable in large measure to the work of the health visitors.

Chapter XVII

THE TREATMENT OF CERTAIN DISEASES IN PUBLIC HEALTH ADMINISTRATION

Tuberculosis

Although the primary aim of preventive medicine is to preserve for each individual the integrity of his physiological life, and to promote all measures tending to maintain it, Public Health in actual practice is concerned in large measure with remedial measures which only come into action when pathological processes have become established. Examples of work which conduces to the primary aim of Public Health are the hygienic care of the expectant mother and of the young child and the provision for them of adequate rest and exercise, of fresh air and bright sunshine, and of food ample in amount, suitably prepared and proportioned, and including the important principles known to abound in butter and cod liver oil, in milk, in fresh fruits and green vegetables, and in wholemeal bread.

Examples of what may be called the secondary work of Public Health, which in present circumstances is still its most urgent work, are seen in the methods adopted in the prevention of the acute infectious diseases and of the more chronic infectious diseases, tuberculosis and venereal disease, especially syphilis. In some of these, especially in smallpox and diphtheria, the human system can be so fortified by the production of artificial immunity as to bring them almost completely within skilled human control. In tuberculosis it is clear that the majority of mankind possess adequate resistance to serious invasion by infection; though even in this special instance much of what is ascribed to increase of resistance—the result of improved hygiene—may in reality be due to decreased dosage of infection by tubercle bacilli. No reasonable hygienist will hesitate to act as if reduction of infection was the main object in view, especially for infants and young children, while making every possible effort by better housing, by adequate food, and by avoidance of over-fatigue and alcoholism, to maintain and improve individual powers of resistance.

In most other infectious diseases, and most importantly in syphilis and gonorrhœa, the sole hope of preventive medicine at present consists in preventing infection by the specific contagium by which each of these communicable diseases is caused. Hence the elaborate official machinery in the Public Health Service for disinfestation of children and adults infested by vermin, for disinfection of infected articles in infectious diseases, for isolation of the infectious sick either at home or in a hospital, and for their treatment as a necessary concomitant of such isolation. It is unnecessary here to discuss the measure of success which efforts in these directions have experienced. It may suffice to say this success has varied greatly in different diseases. The greatest measure of success has been achieved in diseases like typhus and typhoid fever, in which intermediate infection has been controlled, e.g. by purification of specifically polluted water supplies and by cleansing lousy persons as well as by isolating patients suffering from one of these diseases.

In syphilis and gonorrhœa control implies the prevention of contact between infected and non-infected. In tuberculosis whether chief importance is held to attach to prevention of infection or to increase of resistance to infection, there is no difference of opinion as to the great importance attaching to the avoidance of frequent and of large dosed infection; and such avoidance of infection is supremely important for infants and young children. Hence all are agreed that early recognition of pulmonary tuberculosis is very important, followed by sanatorium treatment and practical instruction in hygiene, especially in relation to coughing and expectoration. It is also agreed that institutional treatment or careful separate home treatment with skilled nursing is required in acute exacerbations of tuberculosis and in cases of advanced disease, especially when the patient is bed-ridden.

The provision of special public health machinery for tuberculosis and for venereal disease is justified by the large share of total national sickness and mortality which they cause.

Over 9 per cent. of the total mortality from all causes in England and Wales is returned as due to tuberculosis; and of the total mortality in man at ages 25-45 tuberculosis is responsible for 45 per cent. According to the late Sir William Osler syphilis is more destructive to life than tuberculosis, cancer, or pneumonia, which rank highest in our mortuary tables. These tables show relatively few deaths from syphilis, the medical certificates usually giving the proximal cause of death, not the syphilitic infection which may have been acquired ten or more years before death is caused, e.g. by syphilitic arteritis or general paralysis of the insane. Whatever the exact proportions may be it is probable that tuberculosis, syphilis and alcoholism in the aggregate are responsible for a quarter of the total deaths in this country; and it is noteworthy that nearly all these deaths occur in early life or in adult life, long before the victim has attained an age at which his own efforts can no longer support him in comfort.

Tuberculosis being an infectious disease was made notifiable, each case recognised by the medical attendant being required to be reported to the medical officer of health. This involved a change of policy in the Local Government Board; and partly owing to this, and partly because of the unpreparedness of many local authorities to give the assistance needed for notified cases, the general enforcement of notification was brought about in stages. In 1909 cases of consumption (Phthisis) occurring in poor law practice were made notifiable; in 1911 this obligation was extended to cases in hospital practice; in 1912 phthisis was made notifiable for the general community; and then this obligation was extended to all forms of tuberculosis.

Under the official Regulations framed by the Local Government Board the medical officer of health on receipt of a notification of a case of tuberculosis was required to make such inquiries and take such steps as might be necessary or desirable for investigating the source of infection, for preventing the spread of infection, and for removing conditions favourable to infection. The action taken included *inter alia* :—

(1) Attention to the personal hygiene of the patient, including instruction in the necessary precautions as to coughing and expectoration.

(2) Any assistance needed to ensure for the patient

(*a*) Skilled medical attendance and nursing as required while he is treated at home;

(*b*) Institutional treatment when required;

(*c*) Supplementation of the convalescent patient's funds, when needed, to obviate the necessity for him at once to embark in full-time work; to provide additional bedroom accommodation when needed; and to ensure that the patient and his family are not undernourished or overworked.

(3) Remedial action for any insanitary conditions of the home, such as uncleanliness, dampness, overcrowding; or of the patient's workplace, especially for dusty occupations.

(4) Examination of home "contacts" with the patient.

Scope of Tuberculosis Schemes.—Prior to the general enforcement of notification of tuberculosis in England excellent local work had been done in a relatively small number of areas in direct efforts to control the spread of tuberculosis. This work was in addition to the general measures, which were already being steadily increased, such as improved sanitation, better housing, more satisfactory nutrition, and especially the hospital treatment of a large proportion of advanced and acute cases of tuberculosis. The Report of the last Royal Commission on Tuberculosis appeared in 1911; and although precautions against human infection by tuberculous cows' milk are still very incomplete, the pasteurisation or boiling of milk is more generally practised than in the past.

Local Sanitary Authorities prior to 1911 had power to build sanatoria or otherwise provide institutional accommodation for the treatment of tuberculous patients; relatively little had been done in most areas. In 1911 the Finance Act provided a sum of £1,116,000 for the erection of sanatoria in England and Wales, and this with money provided by local rates, has led to rapid increase in accommodation for the residential institutional treatment of tuberculosis. In England in 1911 local authorities, other than poor law authorities, had about 1,300 beds for the institutional treatment of tuberculosis, while there were 4,200 beds in private sanatoria and voluntary institutions. In 1917 the total available beds numbered 12,441, of which about one-half were provided by local authorities. In 1924 the number of beds similarly approved for the schemes of local authorities had increased to 20,115, of which over 62 per cent. were provided by local authorities.

In 1911 the National Insurance Act was passed

and came into operation in July, 1912. This provided a special "Sanatorium Benefit."

The Departmental Committee appointed to make recommendations as to detailed direct measures against tuberculosis, reported in April, 1912, that any scheme which is to form the basis of an attempt to deal with the problem of tuberculosis should be available for the whole community, and that its organisation should be undertaken by the large local authorities (the councils of counties and county boroughs). These recommendations were at once adopted by the Government, which undertook to provide out of the national exchequer one-half of the net cost of approved local schemes for the treatment of tuberculosis in any member of the community whether insured or not. Local authorities were invited by the Local Government Board at once to prepare schemes for institutional treatment, residential and non-residential, domiciliary treatment remaining in the hands of private practitioners, of poor law doctors, and of doctors engaged in the contract work under the National Insurance Act ("panel doctors"). The last named are in medical charge of the large mass of the wage-earners of the community, comprising roughly one-third of the total population, in so far as their treatment at home is within the capacity of a practitioner of average competence. The anti-tuberculosis schemes proposed for each area comprised:—

(1) The appointment of a tuberculosis officer, usually a whole-time official, who was required to have had special experience in the diagnosis and

treatment of tuberculosis, and who as a rule was an officer in the public health department under the administrative supervision of the medical officer of health, but independent in his clinical work.

(2) The establishment of tuberculosis dispensaries, at which patients were treated, consultations as to doubtful cases held, and contacts examined.

(3) The provision of beds in residential institutions for curable and for acute and advanced cases.

(4) The organisation of arrangements for "following up" and "after-care."

During 1912 and 1913 advance was made in these directions. In 1911 there were 25-30 tuberculosis dispensaries: in 1917 their number had increased to 371. In 1914 the onset of the Great War prevented further development of tuberculosis work and seriously crippled and reduced the efficiency of work already initiated; and this increased as the military demand for medical officers and institutions became greater. Since then the completeness of the organisation has steadily increased, though it cannot yet be said that everything possible is being done, especially in respect of co-operation between private medical practitioners and official agencies.

Sanatorium Benefit.—Under the National Insurance Act the annual sum of 1*s.* 3*d.* was set apart for each insured person as part of a tuberculosis fund. As the result of subsequent bargaining with medical practitioners 6*d.* of this was devoted to the domiciliary treatment of tuberculosis patients (payable on the number of panel patients on each doctor's list, not on the number of his tuberculous patients), the remainder being payable to local authorities who undertook the provision of institutions for the treatment of tuberculous insured patients.

The inextricably interlaced measures for the prevention and the treatment of tuberculosis must necessarily accrue to the whole population. The mistake of the National Insurance Act in ignoring this was soon remedied to the extent that Public Health Authorities were informed that the National Treasury was prepared to pay one-half of the approved expenditure incurred by these authorities in establishing schemes for the treatment of tuberculosis available for the entire population. There remained the fact that insured persons who had paid their weekly quota and were therefore entitled to "Sanatorium Benefit" usually interpreted this as a right to three months' treatment in a Sanatorium. The choice of persons to receive treatment in a Sanatorium lay with Local Insurance Committees appointed under the National Insurance Act, who generally acted on the advice of the tuberculosis officer; but influences other than medical led to the unsatisfactory use of institutional treatment. A large number of patients were sent to and retained in sanatoria for prolonged periods, who might have been adequately treated at home, or who should have been in hospitals. Satisfactory results for sanatorium treatment were not secured under these conditions; and as stated by me elsewhere ("Public Health and Insurance," 1920) "there will probably be no material improvement until the Sanatorium Benefit is withdrawn as a special benefit under the National Insurance Act, and the treatment of tuberculosis becomes an obligatory duty of Public Health Authorities, with a minimum standard of provision to which all must attain."

This was effected in 1921.

The prospect as regards tuberculosis may be summarised in the following statement taken from the work quoted on the preceding page.

"(1) Our knowledge of tuberculosis, if fully applied by combined attack on the disease by all known methods, is adequate to secure a great reduction in its prevalence, if not its absolute abolition.

"This is true, although certain problems respecting tuberculosis still need elucidation, e.g. as to improved methods of treating the diseases, and as to means for increasing individual immunity during exposure to protracted infection.

"(2) Domestic protection is at once practicable against infected cows' milk; and control of this source of infection at its source is also practicable.

"(3) Of the circumstances favouring the development of pulmonary tuberculosis, industrial dust, domestic overcrowding, and defective nutrition of children and young adults are the most potent. More detailed and frequent supervision of factories and workshops is needed, followed by the more general adoption of remedies, which would increase industrial efficiency as well as reduce tuberculosis.

"(4) Tuberculosis is especially a 'bedroom infection.' But improvement in housing is a dual problem, and it is a blunder to assume that improved housing, so long as the healthy and tuberculous sick continue to be housed together, will produce a rapid decline in the prevalence of tuberculosis. Hospital provision for the sick is as necessary as improved general housing."

In addition it must be noted that "(5) No one line of attack against tuberculosis can give complete success. Malnutrition and alcoholism both lower resistance to infection, and a complete campaign against tuberculosis will include greatly increased educational work among the general public, among tuberculosis patients themselves and nurses and others in charge of them, and a great increase in intimate co-operation between what may be described as official and as non-official medicine."

It must not be assumed that measures taken so far have been unsuccessful. The death-rate from tuberculosis has declined steadily without interruption, except in years of epidemic influenza, and this can in large measure be ascribed to the preventive and curative measures which each year extend in scope. The execution of these measures necessitates the steady co-operation of every adult in the community; and it is regrettable that public health authorities and voluntary associations have not pursued educational anti-tuberculosis work with the persistent enthusiasm which its importance deserves. Had the same amount of continuous enthusiasm and driving power being thrown into the anti-tuberculosis campaign which has been evidenced in anti-venereal work our national statistics would almost certainly have displayed a greater improvement than has actually occurred.

Chapter XVIII

THE TREATMENT OF CERTAIN DISEASES IN PUBLIC HEALTH ADMINISTRATION

Venereal Diseases

Past success in the ministration of health has been secured in the main by discovery of the sources of mischief, and by application of measures for their control. This has been chiefly effected by inhibiting the vectors of infection from action, or in one or two instances by the production of artificial immunity in those exposed to attack by infectious disease.

When this exposure is dependent almost entirely on the ability or willingness of the individual to abstain from immoral that is anti-social indulgence, the difficulties of control or prevention are much greater than when, as in typhoid fever or typhus, the fate of the multitude can be beneficially influenced by active preventive work on the part of a few.

Alcoholism and venereal disease are the chief examples of disease caused by directly anti-social conduct; and they happen to be so frequently related that to some extent the action required to reduce one will lessen the other. Together these diseases form the greatest removable obstacles in our midst to health, happiness, and prosperity; and if, in the necessary limitations of this volume

I do not attempt to discuss Alcohol in relation to Public Health, it must still be assumed that this is one of the greatest of public health problems awaiting its complete solution.

The history of attempts to control venereal disease forms an important chapter in social history which cannot be more than briefly indicated here. Behind these diseases, and forming for practical purposes their main source, is the practice of sexual promiscuity, and especially of prostitution, i.e. of commercialised vice; and in the past the public conscience has wavered between complete tolerance of prostitution, attempts to regulate it, and attempts to rid it of its terrible disease-producing capacity. Lecky expressed no more than the truth when he stated that

> "in all nations, ages, and religions, a vast mass of irregular indulgence has appeared which has probably contributed more than any other single cause to the misery and degradation of man."

So far as the attack of the State on prostitution is concerned, it has been largely directed to protecting women and girls, to the prevention of procuration, to an increased age limit for consent, and to the suppression of brothels as inadequately defined by law.

In the 19th Century effort has rather been directed towards attempts to prevent venereal diseases by the sanitation of prostitutes; and it is at this stage that an important exception to the rule that all official health measures should be under unified control appears. The soldiers and sailors of the Army and Navy form a separate body of men aggregated in artificial communities, and most of them unable to marry. In such circumstances much promiscuity was inevitable in the older conditions of long service; though happily it has been lessened in more recent years, owing to shorter service, to improved educational and recreative measures, and to the increasing anti-alcoholic efforts in these forces.

In certain military and naval towns under the Contagious Diseases Acts of 1864, 1866, and 1869, systematic sanitary supervision, including physical examination, of prostitutes was attempted. No great success attended these Acts, and soon serious objection to their continuance arose. On the one hand agitation began which was directed towards extending the operation of the Acts to the civilian population generally. It was realised that the fields of activity of prostitutes and of their consorts could not be limited, and that while it was true that prostitutes flocking to military and naval centres injured terribly the efficiency of the Navy and Army, it was none the less true that the demand created the supply; and that the Acts to be efficient must have a national scope. On the other hand the working of the Acts rendered hospitals necessary which were regarded by the public as being required less for the treatment of the sick than in order to make the prostitute "clean for hire." It was rightly felt that this treatment following in laggard fashion the course of persisting disease did not justify the continuance of compulsory medical examination of prostitutes in the special areas. In short the surveillance and medical examination of prostitutes instituted by these Acts did not succeed in giving " an artificial security to promiscuous fornication " ; the attempted segregation and disinfection of prostitutes failed because it was only able to be applied to a minority of women needing it, and because their male associates were not, and in the main could not in practice be similarly treated.

This is a chief reason why action on these lines must necessarily fail ; and when the Royal Commission on Venereal Diseases was appointed in 1913 to inquire into the prevalence of venereal diseases in the United Kingdom, their effect upon the health of the community, and the means by which these effects could be alleviated or prevented, the proviso was added that " no return to the policy or provisions of the Contagious Diseases Acts of 1864, 1866, or 1869, is to be regarded as falling within the scope of the inquiry." It is significant, further, that the Royal Commissioners, when reporting in February, 1916, expressed the unanimous opinion that in their view " no advantage would accrue from a return to the system of those Acts."

The Royal Commission on Venereal Diseases which sat from November, 1913, to February, 1916, reported in favour of a scheme of universal medical treatment and diagnosis for these diseases, and of educational efforts directed to increasing general knowledge of their dangers and to the attainment of measures tending to secure their moral control.

The prior experience of special hospitals for prostitutes limited to naval and military centres did not contra-indicate the recommendation of provision of treatment for all venereal patients. For this there are several reasons.

(1) Our knowledge of the organisms to which syphilis and gonorrhœa are due has greatly increased. In 1905 the spirochæta pallida was discovered to be the specific organism of syphilis; and later on Noguchi found this organism in the brain of persons dying of general paralysis of the insane. In 1879 Neisser discovered the gonococcus, the infecting organism of gonorrhœa. It thus became possible by microscopic examination to determine the presence of these diseases, when otherwise they might have been overlooked.

(2) Ehrlich's discovery of a new method of treatment of syphilis by salvarsan (and allied arseno-benzol compounds) opened out a greatly increased prospect of cure of syphilitic patients; and furthermore rendered it possible with much greater dispatch than previously to free the patient from his power to infect others.

(3) Added to this came the discovery of the blood test—generally known as the Wassermann test—by means of which the presence of syphilitic infection in the general system is discoverable, and the cessation of this infection can be determined approximately for individual patients.

(4) Under the proposed arrangements for treatment, no social or monetary distinctions were to be

made, the patient was assured of the confidential character of his treatment, and for this purpose the treatment as a rule was to be given in general hospitals, rather than at specially established venereal clinics.

Following on the issue of the Royal Commission's report in March, 1916, the Local Government Board issued regulations and a medical memorandum on the 13th July, 1916, which gave practical effect to the most important recommendations of the Commission.

(1) The Regulations for the first time in history introduced the word "shall" instead of "may," making it obligatory on the councils of county boroughs and counties to prepare schemes for the provision of

(*a*) pathological aids for diagnosis, and

(*b*) the institutional treatment of these diseases.

They were also to be the distributors of gratuitous supplies of arseno-benzol preparations to qualified practitioners for the domiciliary treatment of these diseases.

(2) In view of the extreme importance of administrative action against these diseases the Government undertook to pay three-fourths of approved expenditure incurred by local authorities under headings (1) or (3) which follows. It will be noted that the grants-in-aid were larger than in the case of tuberculosis (page 222); and the rapid provision of facilities for treatment of venereal diseases throughout the country amply justified this exceptionally large grant.

(3) The Regulations provided for expenditure on educational aids to the prevention of venereal diseases. Even so far as treatment and diagnosis are concerned, propagandist work was indicated, in order to secure that the facilities provided should be known to the general public, and to ensure that the facilities for diagnosis and consultation should be utilised to an adequate extent.

In securing this end the National Council for Combating Venereal Diseases has done valuable work; as also in more general educational work on the hygiene of sex and in the wider aspects of social hygiene implicated in the prevention of venereal diseases.

Early in the anti-venereal campaign it was experienced that the success of the efforts being made to induce venereal patients to come for medical treatment was endangered and belittled by the patients' desire for secrecy and by their consequent resort to herbalists and other unqualified persons for treatment. The Royal Commissioners had expressed their view as to the part played by unqualified practice in the perpetuation of these diseases as follows:

> "We have no hesitation in stating that the effects of unqualified practice in regard to venereal diseases are disastrous, and that, in our opinion, the continued existence of unqualified practice constitutes one of the principal hindrances to the eradication of those diseases."

To avert this evil the Venereal Disease Act, 1917, was promoted by the Local Government Board and became law. Its general purport is explained in the following extract from a circular to local authorities issued in September, 1917.

"Section 1 of the Act, which comes into operation in any area to which it is applied by order of the Local Government Board, declares it illegal for anyone, other than a duly qualified medical practitioner, for reward either direct or indirect, to treat any person for venereal disease, or prescribe any remedy for such disease, or give any advice in connection with the treatment thereof, whether the advice is given to the person to be treated or to any other person. As an order of the Board, bringing the section into operation within any area, cannot be made until a scheme for the gratuitous treatment of persons in that area suffering from venereal disease has been approved by the Board and is already in operation, the Council will see the desirability of expediting the completion of the arrangements proposed for dealing with venereal diseases in their area. The Board have recently issued an order, which will come into operation on the 1st November next, applying the provisions of the section to 15 Counties and 21 County Boroughs in which these conditions are already satisfied.

"Section 2 (1) of the Act, which came into operation with the passing of the Act, prohibits advertisements, public notices and announcements (other than advertisements, notices or announcements published by any local or public authority or with the sanction of the Board, or publications sent only to duly qualified medical practitioners or to wholesale or retail chemists for the purposes of their business) with respect to the treatment of venereal disease, or the prescription of remedies therefor, or the giving of advice in connection with the treatment.

"Section 2 (2), which comes into operation on the 1st November next, is directed against the advertisement or recommendation to the public of any so-called remedies for venereal disease by means of any printed papers or hand-bills, or by labels, etc., affixed to or delivered with any packet, bottle, etc., containing any such so-called remedies."

Ere long, owing to the rapid promotion by local authorities of schemes for treatment this Act came into general operation; and it doubtless has assisted greatly in securing skilled treatment for patients who otherwise might have been tempted to resort to quacks.

The Act gives exceptional powers, which have no parallel in other branches of medicine (except more recently in dentistry); and it is evident that such powers could not properly be extended unless Parliament knew that medical provision was available for the general community. This is the case for venereal diseases, and the "warning off" of quacks from what had previously been their favourite subject, is not the least of the factors which is now assisting in reducing the incidence of venereal diseases.

A vast amount of anti-venereal work has been done under these regulations and by means of popular propaganda.

By the year 1918, 127 out of the total 145 local authorities concerned had submitted schemes under the Regulations, providing some measure of treatment for 35 millions out of 36 millions. In March, 1924, the number of treatment centres at work in England and Wales was 184. The figures given in the 5th Annual Report of the Ministry of Health show the extent of this work at the treatment centres in England in the year 1923 :—

Patients dealt with for the first time ..		69,003
Syphilis	22,093	
Gonorrhœa	28,894	
Soft chancre	864	
Not venereal disease	17,152	
Number of attendances		1,527,000
Number of in-patient days		161,000

Without going into details it can be reasonably inferred from the available data that increasing success is being attained in inducing patients to persist in their treatment, and that the total prevalence of the disease is probably decreasing.

The sources of infection, especially of syphilis, have almost certainly been reduced by the educational propaganda, and especially by the prompt and efficient treatment of cases; and the system of gratuitous and confidential treatment of all comers in publicly provided clinics has justified its existence. It needs extension in various directions. Without infringing on the essential principle of privacy, it would be practicable to employ skilled attendants at the clinics to aid in securing uninterrupted attendance of patients, to inquire into family histories, and judiciously to secure the treatment of "contacts." In the investigation of the causation of still-births and in cautious help to families a member of which has acute ophthalmia or has interstitial keratitis or some other evidence of syphilis, there is a field as yet largely untilled, in which invaluable work on medical lines remains to be done. Nor does the above imperfect summary exhaust the possibilities of utility of medical and hygienic work, both in treatment and in instruction, which, although already begun, needs to be multiplied manifold.

But while fully appreciating the great possibilities of extended good work on present lines, there remains a sphere of preventive work, which, although both medical and hygienic in the highest sense of these words, transcends the general scope of present work, and is supremely important.

This is no less than the creation of a higher general conception of sexual morality than is generally held.

Work in this direction not many years ago would have been regarded as totally beyond the scope of official ministration of health; but the giving of aid under the Regulations made in 1916 for educational work in respect of venereal disease renders it possible to promote progress in this direction.

The most efficient means for diminishing sexual promiscuity—the source of venereal diseases—would be found in measures facilitating early marriage for a larger proportion of the total adult population. Public opinion with judicious and continuous effort can be directed towards securing an equally high standard of sexual morality for the two sexes; and the importance of training in early life in the beginnings of self-restraint cannot be exaggerated. The object in respect of each child is the formation of character competent to secure the moral inhibitions which are necessary in a civilised and Christian community.

This sketch of the needs of the community for the control of venereal diseases may be summarised in the following words written by the author in a contribution to the *Hibbert Journal.*

> "The general position embodied and emphasised in the preceding review of this many-sided subject is that complete success in eliminating venereal diseases from the community is to be achieved only by moral means, and that in the final issue the abolition from our midst of one of the greatest scourges of humanity must depend on an increasing realisation, by every parent, teacher, and indeed by all adults, of their responsibility in the training of the young, and on action based on this realised responsibility, beginning in earliest childhood and continuous throughout childhood and youth.
>
> "There is an essential difference between this method of prevention of the most preventable of diseases and the method which is based on instruction in processes of cleanliness and disinfection—competent it may be, but often failing—to render sexual promiscuity safe from the risk of acquiring disease. The moral argument for chastity is alone consistent with the strength, beauty, and joy of an admirable life; though it

is occasionally necessary to deal with the incontinent in tender pitifulness, which is a faint reflection of the care which the mother bestows on her infant before he has learnt to control his excretory functions."

Chapter XIX

MEDICINE AND PUBLIC HEALTH

The extent to which public health administration implies the utilisation of medical skill may be inferred from the aggregate contents of the preceding chapters. While it is true that Public Health is not concerned solely with the special application of physiological and pathological science, over the greater part of the field of work the principles behind public health activities must in the main be based on the sciences of hygiene and medicine.

Local impact between medicine and the public arises in the administrative work of

local sanitary authorities and county councils,
boards of guardians,
local insurance committees,
local education committees,

and in the vast organisations of voluntary hospitals, dispensaries, convalescent homes, etc.

Centrally the Ministry of Health, the Board of Education, and the Home Office are chiefly concerned; and the Privy Council in the work of the Medical Research Council. For present purposes we may leave the medical organisations of the Navy and Army, and of the Pensions Ministry unconsidered.

The extent to which there has been secured co-ordination and fusion of local and central medical official work has been already indicated. It now remains to attempt a conspective view of present arrangements, and to comment on these. This may be attempted from several angles. We may first classify official medical services according to the age of the persons concerned:—

	Central Authorities concerned.	Local Authorities concerned.
The mother during pregnancy	Poor Law Division ... } of Min. of Health Public Health Division } Central Midwives Board } related to Min. of Health	Board of Guardians or Local Health Authority (Mat. and Child Welfare Work)
Childbirth	Insurance Division* ... } of Min. of Health Poor Law Division ... } Public Health Division }	Approved Society Board of Guardians Local Health Authority
Infancy and before compulsory attendance at school	Public Health Division } of Min. of Health Poor Law Division } Board of Education for some children aged 2-5	Local Health Authority Board of Guardians Local Education Authority
Children attending school	Board of Education Public Health Division } of Min. of Health Poor Law Division }	Local Education Authority Local Health Authority Board of Guardians
Aged 14-16	Board of Education (if attending school) Public Health Division } of Min. of Health Poor Law Division } Home Office and Factory Inspectors	{ Local Health Authority { Board of Guardians
Aged 16-70	Insurance Division of Min. of Health (for insured only) Public Health Division } of Min. of Health Poor Law Division } (for all)	Local Insurance Committee { Local Health Authority { Board of Guardians

* Monetary provision only.

The above statement (excepting for the Maternity Benefit) relates only to various forms and sources of official medical aid available in different circumstances.

The persistent confusion of functions and resultant loss of efficiency may be further illustrated by reference to some special branches of medical work.

Laboratory Diagnosis of Disease.

Some limited provision is made in Poor Law Institutions under Boards of Guardians.

The chief provision—but in the main limited to the diagnosis of acute infections and of venereal diseases—is made by Public Health authorities.

Provision was proposed of general pathological facilities in the Budget of 1914 under Public Health Authorities, but was dropped owing to the war.

Domiciliary treatment of disease in general.

By Boards of Guardians for the destitute.
By Local Insurance Committees for one-third of the total population.
By Public Health Authorities for
  certain acute infectious diseases;
  provision of salvarsan for syphilis;
  nursing aid for tuberculosis, measles, etc.

The treatment of tuberculosis.

(*a*) Domiciliary by
  Boards of Guardians,
  Local Insurance Committee (panel doctors),
  Nursing by Public Health Authorities.
(*b*) Institutional by
  Boards of Guardians,
  Public Health Authorities,
  Some Local Education Authorities.

The treatment of venereal diseases.

(*a*) Domiciliary by
Boards of Guardians,
Local Insurance Committee (Panel Doctors partially)

(*b*) Institutional by
Boards of Guardians,
Public Health Authorities.

The provision of midwives and of doctors in consultation.

Local Insurance Committee (indirectly by Maternity Benefit).

Domiciliary and institutional by Boards of Guardians and Public Health Authorities.

Child Welfare Work.

The overlap between Education and Public Health Authorities already noted.

The County Council or the local Sanitary Authority may undertake the public health work.

The multiplicity of overlapping arrangements is further illustrated by the fact that a given medical practitioner in a town may be appointed :—

(1) Part time Medical Officer of Health by the Local Sanitary Authority.

(2) Part time School Medical Officer by the Local Education Authority which may be the County Council and not the Local Sanitary Authority.

(3) District Medical Officer by the Board of

Guardians, whose area commonly does not coincide with that of the Local Sanitary Authority. He may also sometimes be

(4) Public Vaccinator.
(5) Workhouse Medical Officer.
} Appointed by the Board of Guardians.

(6) A panel practitioner under the Local Insurance Committee.

(7) A certifying or Factory Surgeon appointed by H.M. Chief Inspector of Factories, Home Office.

In each of these capacities terms as to payment and duties of the medical practitioner need to be separately negotiated, and the conditions of tenure of office vary greatly.

For Insurance medical work there is a uniform national flat rate of payment; but for nearly all the other appointments enumerated above correspondence with and approval by the poor law or the public health divisions of the Ministry of Health, by the Board of Education, or by the Home Office is required.

The extent to which the medical profession is engaged in official medical work may be inferred from the following figures prepared by me in 1917. The corresponding numbers would now be materially increased, but the general picture is but little altered.

The Medical Services of the State

I. *Number of Medical Officers concerned.*

A. Poor Law.

Workhouse Medical Officers, about (two-ninths whole time officers)	900

District Medical Officers, about .. 3,400
Public Vaccinators, about 3,000

B. Public Health.

For 1,854 sanitary districts and 60 county areas there were

Whole-time Medical Officers of Health, about 300
Assistant Whole-time Medical Officers of Health, about .. 300
Part-time Medical Officers of Health, about 1,100
Tuberculosis Officers 238
Medical Officers of Fever and Smallpox Hospitals, about .. 1,000

C. Lunacy.

There were 350 whole-time medical officers for public lunatic asylums.

D. School Medical Service.

School Medical Officers and Assistant School Medical Officers .. 847
Specialist Medical Officers (part-time or whole-time) 424
(Of the School Medical Officers 261 were also Medical Officers of Health.)

E. Insurance Medical Service.

More than half of the total 26,000 medical practitioners in England and Wales engage in contract practice under the National Insurance Act. Nearly all the district medical officers and two-thirds of the workhouse medical officers are also panel doctors.

Note.—In many instances one officer held several

posts. Over one-third of the medical officers of health were also district medical officers.

The above statement does not include doctors employed as factory certifying surgeons, as police surgeons, or as medical officers under pension schemes or in the Army and Navy. In some particular or other a majority of the medical profession hold some medical post under local or central authorities concerned in the prevention and treatment of disease.

Further light is shown on the extent to which the State, chiefly through Local Authorities, is already engaged in the treatment of disease in the following statement of hospital beds supplied out of rates and taxes. The number provided by voluntary agencies is given for comparison. The figures are derived from the Hospital Return, 1915, and the annual report of the Medical Officer of the Local Government Board for 1913-14.

II. *Number of Hospital Beds provided or rented for the Community by different Authorities.*

	No. of Hospitals.	*No. of Beds.*
A. BY PUBLIC HEALTH AUTHORITIES.		
Fever Hospitals	755	31,149
Smallpox Hospitals	363	7,972
Tuberculosis Sanatoria and Hospitals (England only) ..	287	(*about*) 10,000
Asylums for the Insane ..	109	109,024
Institutions for the Feeble-minded	14	11,559
Total Public Health ..	1,528	169,704

B. By Boards of Guardians.		
Infirmaries and Workhouses ..	700	94,001
Total provided by Public Authorities	2,228	263,705
C. By Voluntary Hospitals.		
General and Special	816	44,983

Thus of the total beds at that period voluntary hospitals provided less than 15 per cent., 85 per cent. being supplied by Public Health and Poor Law authorities. Of the perhaps unexpected excess of official over voluntary hospital accommodation a large proportion consists of asylum beds. If these be excluded from the comparison, the rate-supported beds still form about 78 per cent. of the total.

Some Desiderata of a State Medical Service.

The preceding paragraphs show how vastly the State is committed to responsibility for a large part of the medical work of the community. It is appropriate to consider existing provisions in the light of a number of desiderata, which I cannot express better than in the following sentences which I quote from two memoranda written by me in 1917 and in the early part of the year 1918 on "the medical service of the future."

Extract from 1st memorandum.—Certain principles need to be borne in mind in the organisation of medical work by the State.

(1) Each patient requires to be considered in relation to his circumstances, as to housing, sanitary conditions, and ability to provide nursing and other

aids to recovery. This principle is carried out for tuberculosis, health visitors and nurses undertaking through the public health tuberculosis dispensary organisation the home supervision of insured and non-insured persons as directed by the tuberculosis officer.

Similar arrangements should apply to *all* forms of sickness, as the prospect of recovery depends largely on the domestic conditions under which the patient is attended.

(2) Every case of illness should be considered from the point of view of prevention as well as treatment. Prevention of unnecessary protraction or recurrence of illness is to be aimed at as well as removal of causes of illness. Thus the health visiting and nursing staff is required as well as the doctor.

(3) The doctor in charge of a patient should be in a position to call for a health visitor or nurse as required, and it is important that he should therefore be in touch with the local machinery for public health administration.

(4) So far as a large number of diseases are concerned, there is no distinction between prevention and treatment; as for instance in the prevention of tuberculosis by its treatment under satisfactory conditions, in the rapid prevention of infection of syphilis by treatment by arseno-benzol preparations, and in the prevention of dyspepsia, anæmia, etc. by dental treatment, etc.

Hence the local Public Health Committee, besides the preventive measures under their control, must deal with the treatment of all diseases as well as of the diseases already under their charge. For this purpose the Committee may advantageously be strengthened.

Extract from 2nd memorandum.—The points set out below indicate the goal to be reached. Some of the steps recommended may not be able to be taken at once.

DESIDERATA.

A. *Locally.*

(1) A satisfactory medical service must be both hygienic and therapeutic.

(2) In many respects these overlap, and separation of the two is inimical to the public interest, though the service evidently will comprise a number of different branches.

(3) The chief branches of such a service will be :—

i Research, combined with administration, but with a differentiated special research department.

ii Pathological (including bacteriological), giving all possible facilities in diagnosis and treatment.

iii Public Health. This will comprise subdivisions dealing with the special hygiene of Industries* and of Schools* and with collation and analysis of all available anthropometrical, statistical and medical data for reference and comparisons. The ideal is a complete record of each person's physical and medical history, towards which the child welfare, school, and

* These may need to be kept separate for the present: and many considerations need to be weighed in their transfer.

insurance organisations already furnish detached contributions.

iv Clinical—

(*a*) Institutional. { 1 Residential. 2 Non-residential.

(*b*) Domiciliary.

(4) The clinical service will include

medical attendance,
dentistry,
midwifery,
nursing.

(5) The clinical service will comprise attendance for all forms of sickness, including expert consultative and treatment facilities equal in essential respects to those now available for the rich.

(6) The present local medical services of the post office and of the police will be included in the general service.

(7) All influences, monetary or other, tending to inhibit the full use of the medical service to the extent indicated by the medical needs of the patient, must be abolished. This should apply equally to domiciliary and to institutional treatment.

(8) All the above medical duties should be controlled locally by a single local authority. This would be the county council or county borough council and urban district council with a population of at least 20,000. For the last named certain limitations will be required.

B. *Centrally.*

The fulfilment of the above desiderata implies the bringing together under the supervision and control of the Ministry of Health of:—

(1) The preventive and clinical work of county councils and sanitary authorities (general public health, hospital provision, care of lunatics and feeble-minded, maternity and child welfare work, treatment of tuberculosis and of venereal diseases, etc.).

(2) The medical work and the care of children, aged persons, feeble-minded and insane, now undertaken by Boards of Guardians.

(3) The medical work of the Pensions Ministry.

(4) The medical work of the Ministry of National Service.

(5) The administration of the Medical Benefit and the Sanatorium Benefit under the National Insurance Commission; possibly also of the Maternity Benefit.

(6) The medical work of the Board of Education for children under 5 not in attendance at school; and possibly its other medical work later.

It will be important also that:—

(7) The supervisory work of the Privy Council in relation to the General Medical Council, the Central Midwives Board and Pharmacy should be under the same central control. So far as the General Medical Council is concerned, this implies an Imperial as well as a National Ministry of Health.

There can be no difference of opinion as to the incompleteness of the medical service supplied under the Insurance Act. It supplies what the patient apart from an organised medical service could more easily obtain than any other medical need. The services most lacking for the insured and for a large share of the non-insured are :—

(1) A medical service, contributory or non-contributory according to the means of each family, which will supply

Laboratory facilities for diagnosis and in treatment, including access to Rontgen ray facilities;

Consultant facilities in cases of dubious diagnosis;

Consultant facilities in special diseases of the eye, nose, throat, etc.

Such a service, were the separate organisation of poor law medical work to cease, could commonly be arranged at and round poor law infirmaries, or at dispensaries connected with these.

(2) Hospital treatment for the rapidly increasing proportion of patients needing institutional treatment is urgently required and given available poor law beds could be supplied on a greatly increased scale. The increasing need for hospital treatment is a natural result of the great advances in surgery, and of the need in non-surgical cases for the special consultative services which are accessible in a well-organised hospital.

Some of the additional means by which this hospital service may be secured are mentioned later.

(3) A medical service cannot be regarded as satisfactory which does not give in essential matters, e.g. in the provision of consultants and expert facilities equal provision for poor and rich alike; though graduated payment may be required from one and none from the other.

(4) There is needed an extension of the already large provision for skilled nursing, especially domiciliary nursing, so that every practitioner may be able to call for a nurse for his poorer patients. Treasury Grants of half the total expenditure for nurses are already given for cases of puerperal fever, of ophthalmia neonatorum, of measles, whooping cough, pneumonia and poliomyelitis, and diarrhœa; and half the salaries of health visitors and tuberculosis nurses employed by public health authorities are paid by the Ministry of Health.

The preceding statement of requirements emphasises the need of co-operative medical work, for it is impossible for one doctor to be skilled in all branches of medical work; but the adoption of the measures recommended above is not inconsistent with continuance and extension of the work of the general practitioner, who may be regarded as the keystone in the arch of medical provision. In the future the preventive possibilities of his access to patients will be more fully realised; and he will be the family guide giving advice at intervals which will prevent disease or lead to its discovery in its beginnings when prevention and treatment become identical.

The growth of a medical service such as is adumbrated in preceding paragraphs must necessarily be gradual and somewhat slow. Considerations of financial ability necessarily come into the problem; though means for prevention and adequate treatment of disease always cost less than uncontrolled disease. If it be fully appreciated that the present medical ministration of health for the community does not suffice for the public health, and that additional and more perfect provision is needed for all classes in the community, then measures of the right character will begin to be adopted.

In my view the most urgently needed provision, and the one which outside public provision there is the greatest difficulty in obtaining is that of

Laboratory Facilities for diagnosis and treatment.—For tubercle and venereal diseases, and for typhoid fever, diphtheria and a few other diseases free pathological examinations are now commonly provided in all sanitary areas. This subject was reviewed by me in a report (Appendix A. No. 9) printed in the Report of the Medical Officer of the Local Government Board, 1912-13. It was shown that official pathological work was far from complete, and details were given of the valuable pathological work being done by many voluntary hospitals, covering a much wider field of disease than that hitherto compassed by local authorities. The conclusion reached was that "in order that a satisfactory service may be secured throughout the country, facilities for work similar to that now being done in hospitals will need to be offered to medical practitioners generally." The details of a scheme to this end (including physical and chemical as well as pathological laboratory facilities) were worked out, and in the Budget for 1914 a large Treasury Grant was promised for this purpose; but the Great War which followed prevented the adoption of the scheme. This provision, available for all classes of medical practice, still remains an important lack in the scientific treatment of disease.

Schemes for developed Medical Aid.—A report of

the Consultative Council on Medical and Allied Services to the Ministry of Health (Lord Dawson, Chairman) was issued in 1920. It sets out in some detail arrangements for health centres and a domiciliary service for the entire community which, were they suitably dovetailed into the general scheme of public health administration, would assist in the building up of an adequately correlated system of medical help for the community. Allusion may be made to an earlier admirable effort of Dr. Middleton Martin, County Medical Officer of Health of Gloucestershire, to bring into action a plan of medical services for the whole county, including primary health centres, and utilisation of cottage and other hospitals, with a Teaching Hospital in Bristol, and further consultation centres at Cheltenham and Gloucester. The development of such a system beyond the treatment of school children presents great difficulties in present circumstances.

In actual experience in England progress is always step by step, and the solution of the hospital problem is being sought in tentative local efforts, to which a brief reference may be made.

(1) The use of poor law infirmaries for paying patients on a limited scale has already been mentioned.

(2) In Sheffield an admirable scheme has been organised. A very large proportion of its industrial firms join with their men in contributing at the rate of 1*d.* in the £1 of annual wages, the sum thus collected being distributed among the voluntary hospitals of the city and forming a large part of

their total income. Other towns and particular firms have moved in the same direction.

(3) A Hospital Saving Association has been formed which invites people within the hospital income limits to subscribe 3*d.* weekly which will ensure for them and their families any hospital treatment that is needed. The weekly sum is often partly paid by employers. In this and all other schemes it is indispensable that the hospital authority should be quite free to reject or receive patients on medical grounds alone.

(4) The British Provident Association (Hon. Sec., Dr. Gordon Dill) is intended to meet the needs of a wider public. The cost of maintenance of an in-patient in a metropolitan hospital amounts to about £5 a week, a sum which is a serious tax even on middle class people, though it can easily be met under an insurance scheme. This Association, for an annual subscription of 21*s.* for single persons, of 31*s.* 6*d.* for a married couple, and of 42*s.* for a family, provides such hospital and consultative help as may be needed.

(5) Many Approved Societies under the National Insurance Act have contributed some of their surplus funds to voluntary hospitals.

(6) Following on the war, subscriptions to voluntary hospitals fell seriously, and in order to tide over the temporary difficulty the Government made a grant of half a million sterling, to be distributed on a defined basis to voluntary hospitals. It should be mentioned also that many voluntary hospitals receive payment from local authorities for work done for school children, for cases of tuberculosis,

of venereal disease, etc. This does not necessarily imply a future absorption of the voluntary into officially supported hospitals. There is much to be said for the continuance of independent voluntary hospitals, which will accept payment for patients on an insurance basis, while continuing their charitable work for the impoverished.

There necessarily arises the question as to whether the "Medical Benefit" under the National Insurance Acts should continue to be administered as at present. The "Sanatorium Benefit," providing special treatment for insured tuberculous patients has already been abandoned; for it meant that insured persons were paying (in part) for what in well organised sanitary areas non-insured persons were receiving gratuitously. This was a necessary result of the fact that tuberculosis being a communicable disease, its control is a problem of Public Health. But is not every disease a problem of Public Health?

It is true that some diseases are amenable to the measures coming within the range of present Public Health Administration, and some are not so amenable. But even such diseases as heart disease or cancer may be regarded as coming within the range of public health administration. I do not now refer to the possibilities of preventing these diseases: the possibility for instance of preventing heart mischief by attacking morbid tonsils, and still more by preventing syphilis; or the possibility of preventing cancer by stopping chronic sources of local irritation, whether they be lesions of the cervix uteri, excessive smoking, the drinking of spirits, gall stones, or other agents. Apart from such undeveloped possibilities of prevention there is *the more general application of skilled diagnosis and of early and adequate treatment as a means of preventing the phenomena of developed disease.* This is supremely important for heart disease in children; it is equally so for early lesions suspected to be malignant.

Curtailed illness and shortened convalescence are among the greatest gifts of modern surgery in a large range of morbid conditions; and the public as a whole are vitally concerned in the adequate supply of these gifts, not only for humanitarian reasons, but also in order to increase industrial and social efficiency, and to prevent the burden of dependent sickness.

There is much to be said therefore for the abolition of the Medical Benefit of the Insurance Act, and its merging into a wider scheme which will include the dependents of the insured, and some others of nominally larger incomes, who equally require the adequate medical help which can be supplied under an extended insurance scheme. Such a scheme would need to be elastic enough to ensure equally good medical aid for those unable to pay insurance premiums. That eventually progress will be made in this direction, I have no doubt; though delay is likely in view of financial considerations.

Chapter XX

PUBLIC HEALTH AS A CAREER

Summary of Preceding Chapters

Not infrequently the practical question is asked as to the possibility of Public Health as a life career. It may be hoped that a perusal of the preceding chapters will have stimulated readers to enlist in this service. The service is so multifarious that all may find scope for their help.

We may first recall the enormous need for voluntary unpaid workers which is ever pressing. The greater part of such voluntary work, as already indicated, is being done in parliament, and on the local councils of county and borough councils, of education committees, of boards of guardians, and of other official and semi-official bodies directly concerned in public health work. For those possessed of private means, and imbued with the desire to better the conditions of life for their fellows, it would be difficult to name a more satisfying mission in life. To undertake it implies a willingness to come into the "rough and tumble" of opposed activities, to submit to the vagaries of popular electorates, and to be ready to engage in much drudgery as well as to aid in the solution of difficult but vitally interesting social problems. But given this willingness the rewards are great, and the work is essentially Christian. Similar remarks apply to the vast spheres of voluntary unofficial work, which have influence on the public health. This work oft-times forms the necessary preliminary to official work, and even when there is official work of similar character, the voluntary worker has ample scope in filling up gaps and in promoting the higher efficiency of official efforts.

For those who look to work bearing on public health as a career, first mention must be made of the investigator. It will have been evident that further advances in many directions are prevented only by the deficiency of knowledge of the causation of the evils to be combated. The increasing grants for investigation in preventive medicine, and the probability that ere long there will be a vast extension of public health pathological work (see p. 255) call for skilled investigators in many branches of physics and physiology as well as in the pathology of individual diseases. The great need is a larger army of investigators; and happily the possibility of a livelihood from such research work is now brighter than it has hitherto been. In this work it is not only the doctor of medicine who is required; but also those trained in collateral branches of science, from whom may come the chief light on further progress in the prevention of disease and in the elevation of the general standard of health.

In the medical department of public health work there is a steady though relatively small demand for medical practitioners who (page 36) have become diplomates in public health, and are therefore eligible for appointment as medical officers of health.

The duties of these officers and the conditions of their appointment, including the methods of obtaining a special diploma in public health, have already been detailed (page 40). With increased security of tenure of office, thus safeguarding the conscientious worker against dismissal for excessive zeal in discharge of his duties, the medical officer of health can now safely regard public work as a career for life. When a contributory system of pensions tenable after the age of 65, or earlier in the event of permanent disablement, has been accepted by all local authorities (page 38), the conditions of efficient service and of recruital from the best elements in the medical profession will be fulfilled; if, in addition, the salaries given compare not unfavourably with the earnings of competent medical practitioners. For some time past there has been improvement in this respect, although some local authorities have not yet realised the extent to which this condition is wrapped up with the public interests. At present a county medical officer of health may expect to begin work at a salary of about £1,200, the medical officer of health of a town with a population of 200,000 at about £1,300, salaries being graded upwards and downwards according to population, but with a minimum which for a whole-time chief officer should not go below £800 or £900. Assistant medical officers and medical officers of special departments (child welfare, tuberculosis, venereal disease) are paid on a somewhat lower scale; but in view of the fact that promotion to a chief position can only occur in a minority of instances it is greatly in the public interest that these professional salaries should be adequate.

Public analysts are required for all areas. They must be Fellows of the Institute of Chemistry. Emolument is usually according to the number and character of the samples of food and drugs that are analysed.

Chief sanitary inspectors in large towns can obtain a salary of £450 to £500; and district inspectors, inspectors of foods, and inspectors under the Factory and Workshops Acts about £250 to £300. These officers are expected to possess special sanitary knowledge, which has been tested in examination by such bodies as the Royal Sanitary Institute and the Sanitary Inspectors Board.

The work of Health Visitors has already been discussed in Chapter XVI, and the outline of the present conditions as to their appointment has also been indicated. For socially-minded women, who are nurses, but who are keenly interested in the prevention of disease rather than in the treatment (nursing) of the sick, the position of a health visitor offers great attractions. The good that can be effected by a tactful, sympathetic and well-trained health visitor in the families of the people is almost unlimited. Her work may consist solely in the domestic visitation of mothers and infants, and this work is responsible in no small degree for the remarkable decline in infant mortality in recent years (page 71). Or she may specialise in visitation of cases of tuberculosis, or in the work of a "school nurse"; or her work may be made more general, by combining all these and allied duties. The arguments for and against specialisation are indicated on page 215. The salary obtainable by a health visitor may be from £215 to £255. The majority receive round about £200, which is not adequate in present circumstances of life.

To sum up. In the earlier chapters we have shown the gradual unfolding and expansion of public health work culminating in the formation of the Ministry of Health, which represented an important advance in the unification of the ministration of health. In these chapters there is seen the ebb and flow of opinion as to the relative powers of local and central health authorities; and a careful study of these oscillations in opinion and practice has valuable lessons for the future. The study of the steadily improving machinery for securing the public health is also most instructive. Both in factory work and in general public health work, as we have seen, improvement has been secured largely through the work of paid officials possessing special knowledge, whose reports have shed the necessary light on sanitary and social evils, and have impelled legislative and administrative control.

The chapters on the public health work of the Factory Department of the Home Office and of the Board of Education show that recent advances towards central unification of public health work have been only partial. How far further central unification is called for need not be further discussed here; but the contents of the chapters dealing with administration as to Destitution and as to

Insurance against sickness show that there is urgent need, in the interest of efficiency, for the reforms of Poor Law administration which theoretically form a fairly generally agreed policy, and for revision of the local administration of insurance. The formation of the Ministry of Health was the preliminary step to the general reform and redistribution of the work of Boards of Guardians, of Local Sanitary Authorities, and of Insurance Committees which is still lacking. These reforms will carry with them a more complete knitting together of the various local measures for medical and hygienic supervision of and aid to members of the community at every stage of life, and the gradual extension of these measures. The final chapters attempt to demonstrate that the general welfare of the community is more dependent on the prompt and efficient treatment of disease, on its prevention, and on the enhancement of the general standard of health secured by measures of public health and personal hygiene, than on any other conditions.

> "There is little doubt" said the late Dr. Rivers, "that when the history of the medicine of to-day comes to be written, the greatest achievement will not be found in the operative procedures, the antitoxins and the glandular extracts which bulk so largely in the estimation of the profession and of the laity, but in the systematic development of the public health service in our own country, and the still more striking measures by which the tropical regions of the earth are being made available for the service of mankind in general."

INDEX

INDEX

For Product Safety Concerns and Information please contact our EU representative GPSR@taylorandfrancis.com
Taylor & Francis Verlag GmbH, Kaufingerstraße 24, 80331 München, Germany

www.ingramcontent.com/pod-product-compliance
Lightning Source LLC
LaVergne TN
LVHW011118300926
849160LV00008B/429

* 9 7 8 1 1 3 8 9 0 5 2 7 6 *